Morales Method®

Core Integration Therapy:

A unique approach to Structural Integration Bodywork

Revised edition

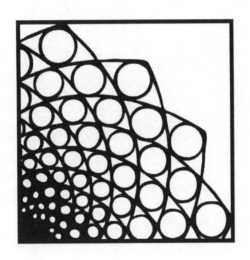

Marty Morales, founder of The Morales Method® of Manual
Therapy & Body Conditioning, Certified Advanced Rolfer™, MBA

illustrations by Xiley Roscher

ISBN: 1500660442
ISBN-13: 978-1500660444

DEDICATION

I dedicate this book to my family and to my students and clients; past, present, and future. You are my greatest teachers.

CONTENTS

ACKNOWLEDGMENTS

Marty Morales the bodyworker would not be where he is today without the guidance, teachings and friendship of Art Riggs. Art took me under his wing and encouraged me to pursue training at The Rolf Institute® of Structural Integration. He still encourages me to this day! At The Rolf Institute I received some of the best training and learned a beautiful craft from teachers such as Jon Martine, Kevin McCoy, Monica Caspari, and the renowned Jan Sultan. Their training created the spark that made me think of this way of working. For Art Riggs and The Rolf Institute I am ever grateful and respectfully acknowledge the lineage of this work.

1 INTRODUCTION

This book is about exploring a different way of thinking and working with regards to Structural Integration (SI). In it we will explore current ways of working and also re-visit innate knowledge and see how it relates to Structural Integration. What is Structural Integration? According to the International Association for Structural Integrators (IASI), "Structural Integration (SI) is a somatic practice utilizing fascial manipulation, awareness, and movement education. It is practiced in an organized series of sessions and individual sessions within a framework designed to restore postural balance and functional ease by aligning and integrating the body in gravity. Structural Integration is based on the work of Dr. Ida P. Rolf.".

Dr. Rolf's way of seeing life has influenced countless people (either as clients or as practitioners) around the world. From her way of working came the Rolf Institute of Structural Integration which has influenced and inspired many other schools and modalities, including this one.

This book is intended to be used during Morales Method® workshops and it helps practitioners gain knowledge in body reading and working with clients in a way that will help them get out of pain, improve their posture, and help them explore a different way of being in their bodies. The first chapters will deal with body reading and assessment and the subsequent chapters will deal with the philosophy of the Morales Method® Core Integration (referred to as MMCI). Included in this book is a review of certain myo-fascial techniques that are commonly used in this type of work. Keep in mind that Morales Method® Core Integration deviates from the classic Structural Integration philosophy in that its aim of achieving results does not preclude it from adapting and integrating other modalities and it will seek to get the client out of pain before moving on to working in a series and integrating the whole system. **Just as this system keeps evolving, so will this book.** Fascial manipulation and movement education are not the sole resources of MMCI.

At the time the first edition of this book was written, it was the only Structural Integration book to include a protocol (classically referred to as the 'recipe') and to show how the protocol is worked. Some practitioners may believe that it is enough to follow this book and from there they will learn how to perform Structural Integration, but it's not that easy. Training must be done by a practitioner under the guidance of a qualified instructor in order to fully understand and acquire the nuances of this work. Only then can Structural Integration be fully 'grocked'.

List of Structural Integration Schools, as of 2014 from www.theiasi.net
1. Australian School of Applied SI & Somatic Studies
2. Holographic Touch
3. Czech Association for Structural Integration
4. The Guild for Structural Integration
5. Hellerwork® International
6. Institut fur Strukturelle Korpertherapie
7. Institute for Structural Integration
8. Institute of Structural Medicine
9. International Professional School of Bodywork
10. International School of Structural Integration
11. Kinesis Myofascial Integration – KMI
12. Mana Integrative Therapies
13. New School of Structural Integration
14. Northwest Center for Structural Integration
15. The Rolf Institute® of Structural Integration
16. SI Australia
17. SOMA Institute of Neuromuscular Integration®
18. Structural Innovations – SI Program

In 2003, after making a drastic career change, I graduated from massage school and started on a new career path. I was working as a massage therapist and providing relaxing massages. In 2004 I took a class with Art Riggs and my work changed to more deep tissue therapeutic work. I liked the results I was getting by helping people get out of pain. Over the next couple of years I came to realize that there was something missing in my practice. I was pretty good at helping folks get out of pain but their pain kept coming back and I had a hunch things weren't as simple as, "it hurts them there so that's where I work". In 2007, after looking at all my options, I decided to receive the Rolfing® ten series (at the suggestion of Art Riggs) and from there I realized there was a whole other paradigm to bodywork and decided to pursue training at the Rolf Institute.

In 2008 I graduated (training in Boulder, Colorado and in Brazil) as a Certified Rolfer™ and started to provide Rolfing® tens session series. Over the next couple of years I started to play with how I was working with the Rolfing series. I started to add in other things I learned, stripping off things that were not working for me, and blended it all to eventually have a series of sessions that appealed to me. I saw how these changes were having a positive effect on my clients. Slowly but surely I was creating my own way of Structural Integration. The philosophy remained but I had brought in aspects of the stages of motor development in babies and had two distinct ways of working on my client's tissues. The exploration of this new way of Structural Integration is the subject of this book.

When it comes to helping our clients, we sometimes walk a fine line in working with structure. This type of work will utilize models of body reading that use ideal angles, planes, and lines but moving someone towards an ideal plane or angle doesn't necessarily equate to their pain relief. Many studies have shown this. With MMCI we understand this and that meeting our objective doesn't always coincide with making sure a leg rotates the ideal number of angles or that an arm can abduct in its ideal full range of motion. We use these methods as a way to give the client a possible better option of being but don't follow degrees of freedom as dogma. To put it another way and to paraphrase Ida Rolf, we work this way because it's "what we can get our hands on".

Rolfing® and other forms of SI usually work as a series of sessions. With MMCI we do not simply imitate the same Rolfing® series of sessions but instead explore a different perspective and approach to Structural Integration that follows its own type of series. We also seek to continue to question the work and to bring in modern thinking and perspectives into the fold. Eventually, this work is able to help the practitioner envision a series of sessions that takes into account the client's needs at that current point in time and create a series of sessions based on those needs. The practitioner at some point has the freedom to be creative and 'play' with the process to create their own series of sessions. Before a practitioner can improvise, a structure must first be followed and adhered to in order to help the practitioner understand MMCI.

If it hasn't been clear enough, I will re-emphasize that this book is not intended to teach Rolfing®. I encourage any bodyworker who wants to learn Rolfing® and become a Certified Rolfer™ to attend The Rolf Institute® of Structural Integration. The Rolf Institute is the origin of this type of work and their program is top notch, home to some of the best instructors in the world with a deep and rich lineage. The intention here is to offer a different approach to Structural Integration that is derived from the original lineage and has been 'field tested' in the lab of my private practice.

Gravity and how people relate in gravity has always been a key influence in the original works of Structural Integration but the stages of motor development in babies has a strong influence in MMCI. Here, we strive to reinforce the client's original pattern that blossomed as they developed as babies, from lying down to vertical position, especially in walking/movement. We do this because our clients mostly move about during their day, they aren't in a static position. A client doesn't spend their waking hours (hopefully) lying down but usually standing, walking, or sitting, so any body-reading and bodywork we do looks at the whole client and they developed in their world. Being able to assess your client and 'read' their 'dynamic posture' is key in determining where to work first, which is an important question we ask ourselves. This is not an easy task. I believe being able to body read the way Structural Integrators do is very much an art form that has puzzled many researches seeking to put it 'in a box'. Once understood however, it can be a very rewarding way to work.

As we do Structural Integration (SI), we explore different ways of reading body posture and use different assessment techniques to verify our findings. It's important to understand that although we are looking at our clients' bodies with the intention of giving them relief from pain and tension, we need to remember that an ideal posture does not necessarily equal pain relief or comfort. As famed SI instructor, Monica Caspari says, "happiness is more important than perfection. Through proper assessment and body reading, we strive to implement tools that will equate to functional ease, not necessarily structural perfection.

> ## "Happiness is more important than perfection"
> ## Monica Caspari

Do we strive to change our client with MMCI? Do we force our will into their system? Or instead, could we give them the option or ability to move along a spectrum of movement rather than stay in a new fixed place in a spectrum? This new option where they are able to move can now be seen as a new 'resource' for the client, a place they can draw from in their lives. As a practitioner of MMCI, we strive to give our clients more resources so they have the ability to adapt to different situations. This work is not about changing someone. Instead, it is about offering up different options of being in the body that may benefit a person when need be. Being able to move along a spectrum gives the client more adaptability in daily life.

Structural Integration provides options for movement along a spectrum

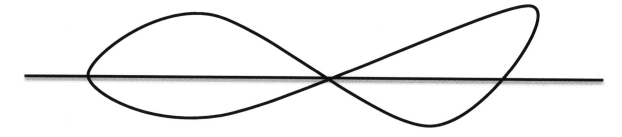

NOTES

I'm often asked, by clients and by students, "So, will the changes stay with me forever?"
This is a legitimate question and it's important for the practitioner to understand the client is coming at this question from a standpoint of: I want to get the most from my time/energy/money investment. Permanence, as I've seen in my practice is not something we seek to stay in but rather something we seek to *move in*. A client, once they've been shown another way of moving/walking/being through this work, can now have that option of being in their system. In modern perspectives it is thought that the practitioner has affected the client's nervous system to accept another way of moving/being. Now that the client has that 'option', they are free to move about within a spectrum of movement as previously shown. This ability to move from one resource to another is what can lead a client to prefer one way over another. Not only that, the client can recall a resource almost at will. This ability is to have a resource, prefer a resource, and be able to recall a resource is the state of permanence we as practitioners are often asked about. I often tell the client it's up to them whether or not they accomplish 'permanence' with the caveat that permanence is fluid.

Many body reading styles look at bodies in static position. When we look at the different postures in our clients, it's easy to look and say one area is tight or another area needs work. Looking at people in static is a good beginning but we should also look at people in movement. Why? In movement we can see how the relationship between different body parts/territories play out during the client's functional activity. For example, a high shoulder can show you its relationship to a misaligned toe if the client is having to lift up their shoulder to compensate for the lack of flexion/extension in the toe, or a sideways curve can be evidently related to a tight psoas. It's very easy to get caught up in the static way of reading and assessing but I suggest you incorporate movement/walking in your readings and assessments to make sure your work becomes more functional and alive. The difference between static body reading and body reading in walking/movement is the difference between a boxer only hitting a bag and a boxer hitting a bag AND sparring. Only one method is good but it is not as 'alive' as practicing the art in function.

Before I go into body reading in movement, I usually get the body reading juices flowing by looking at static posture. In the following figures, which muscle groups would you say are possibly short/tight in the following situations:

NOTES

1. A combination posture of kyphosis and lordosis
2. An extreme lordosis posture
3. A more neutral/natural posture
4. A 'military' straight back type of posture
5. A kyphosis prone posture

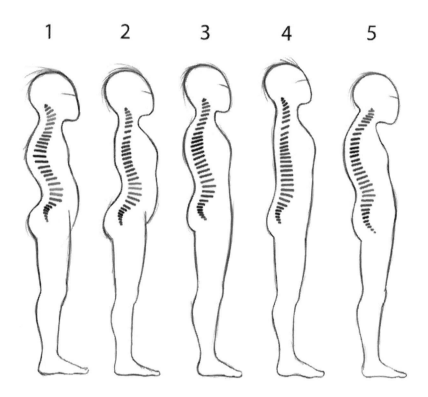

How do these different postures relate to gravity? If you were to work on clients with these different postures, where and how would you work?

As mentioned, this approach is not the root of MMCI but it's a good place to start when starting to body read. One thing to notice when looking at static posture are the arms (notice the arms were not included in the above drawings). The arms can affect and be affected by the rest of the body. In body reading the arms can highlight other areas that need focus.

When doing body reading in movement it's important to understand that simply knowing anatomy is not the solution to body reading and neither is being adept at kinesiology. When body reading for MMCI we move along this process: understanding anatomy, then kinesiology, then understanding functional movement. We strive to define what's happening with our client not just from what's happening with a soleus or a trapezius for example but what is happening in the client's movement that may involve territory that includes soleus or trapezius. Notice I said, 'territory' and not the actual muscle. The reason for this is because functional movement is not solely the property of muscle. Functional movement, as we have learned from the works of Robert Schleip (see www.fasciaresearch.de for numerous articles on the matter) involve muscle and fascia.

One of the biggest differences with MMCI and other forms of bodywork is the way we see what core is and where it's located. Here, we revisit what we have previously believed as 'core'. Many have believed that the body's 'core' involves only the abdominal area. If we look at how we describe the core of an apple, we see that it involves the entire cylindrical inner part of it. This is how we will see the body's core in MMCI. It will involve the abdominal area but also include a cylindrical inner part that incorporates territory taken up by many types of tissue, the spinal column being one of them.

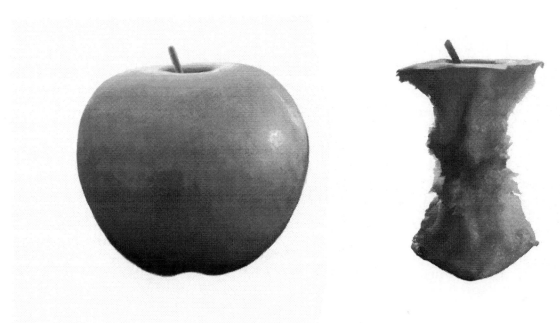

The Core of an Apple, as a reflection of our own human 'inner core'

When I work with a client I see their body having a core that resembles this similar column. The column goes from the bottom of the pelvis to the top of the head. I see movement along different planes of the column (including rotational movement) and in the areas that extend away from the column (the appendages). To me, this central part is the core. What other systems, anatomical or metaphysical, follow this same thought-path? We have the entire spinal column of the skeletal system, the endocrine system, the energy path of Kundalini, and the chakra system.

In the next chapter we will discuss certain areas we can look at in the body when we see our clients walk in order to body read and assess.

The areas we'll discuss are by far not the only areas to look at but for those of us starting out on this path, it takes us in a great direction. The way I've taught this method for years is to give the practitioner the understanding that although our goal is to be able to see the client as a whole system, it's not easy to start body reading that way. Instead, we need to deconstruct the system into small understandable parts and then move on from there to be able to put the parts together and understand the relationships between the parts.

In walking, we look at how several parts of the body move/don't move along the three major planes and also in rotation. They include:

1. Toes
2. Talus
3. Calcaneus
4. Arches (medial and lateral)
5. Navicular & cuboid
6. Knee joint
7. Femur
8. Greater trochanter
9. Pelvis/sacrum
10. Spinal column and thoraco-lumbar junction
11. Gleno-humeral joint
12. Scapula
13. Humerus
14. Lower arm, hands, and head.

What we do is look at these parts in relation to how they move within specific planes and how they articulate, either freely or with restriction. These restrictions could be either myo-fascial, bone, viscera, or nerve related.

When we look at planes we look at them in this order: First sagittal, then coronal, then transverse, and finally rotational movement. We look at how these planes relates to the human body along the vertical axis. The reason for this order is because we mimic the order in which we develop movement in the early stages of motor development. These stages of development have particular themes that interact with the previously mentioned planes.

NOTES

BODY PLANES

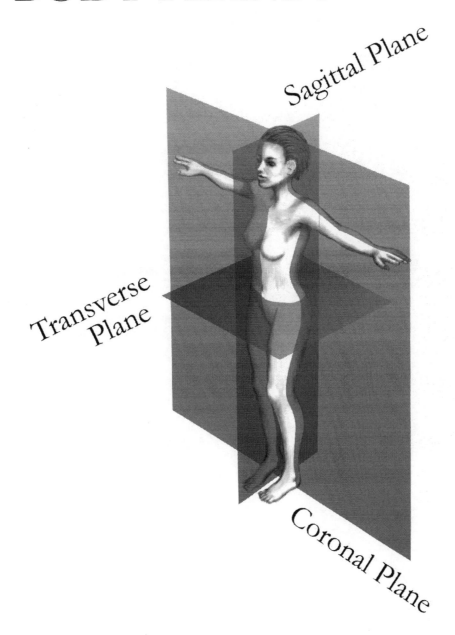

Sagittal Plane

Transverse Plane

Coronal Plane

The Stages of Motor Development

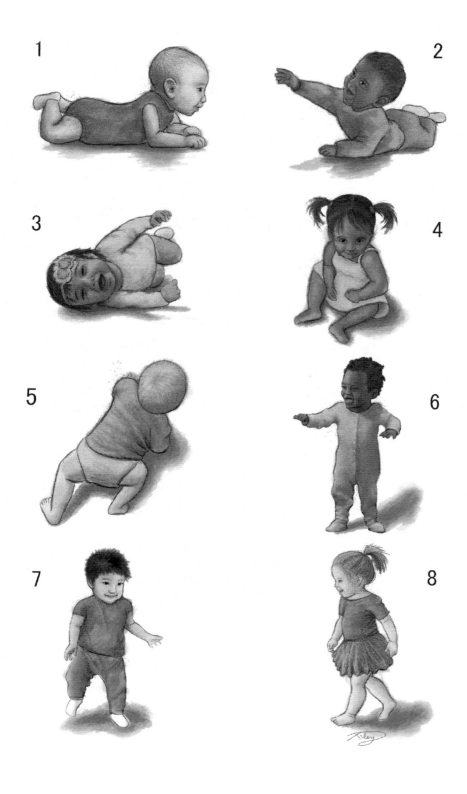

In the beginning of our motor development, we bring our head up as we start to create a cervical curve, as seen with baby #1. This is part of our first movements, a theme of movement along the sagittal plane. The sagittal plane is then our Primary Plane. Eventually we create extension in our lumbar spine and we lift ourselves up from our arms and elbows, almost like the yoga 'cobra pose'. Just like baby #2. This continuing movement in extension, continues the theme of movement along the sagittal plane. Then comes what we'll call the 'rollover'. At first glance when you see a baby do this move we mistake it for rotation of the spine when in actuality what is happening is the baby (when in supine, moving to prone position) is flexing their lower body (at the hip joint) in order to let gravity bring them to prone position. When in prone position, the baby will extend their arm and spine in order to again bring themselves off balance again and then 'roll' into supine position. Baby #3 is displaying flexion that will bring them into prone position. This movement continues the theme of flexion/extension which stays within the sagittal plane. Can you see how important the sagittal plane is? It's so important three major stages of motor development continue to reinforce movement along the sagittal plane.

Eventually we learn to sit as does baby #4. This sets the stage for movement along a different plane. As we develop into our next stage, we as babies will do the back and forth side-bending action in our spine that, when combined with movement of our arms and legs, propels us forward in a crawling manner, just like baby #5. Two major things happen here in this stage:

1. The side-bending action of our spine in crawling creates movement along the coronal plane

2. The action of our arms and legs are in contra-lateral motion. This means that when the left knee moves forward, the right arm moves forward and vice versa. Can you see the movement along the coronal plane in baby #5?

When we start to stand, we again set the stage for movement in another plane. Baby #6 is figuratively and literally about to take a very important step! As baby #7 begins to take his first steps, they are not the refined steps taken from an adolescent or adult. Instead, they are a bit more of a 'waddle'. Some babies walk with their arms up in the air when they start to 'waddle'. In this stage, the baby's pelvis moves in a transverse or lateral motion, from side to side. This is when the transverse plane comes into the picture. Walking becomes more refined and finessed with baby #8. There is less of the waddle and more contra-lateral movement of arms and legs (crawling set the stage for that). Another thing that starts to happen is start to see the integration of all these planes of movement in the spine. When you combine sagittal, coronal, and transverse planes we get rotation and rotation is what starts to happen in small amounts in the baby's spine when they walk like baby#8. We have just revealed how the planes of movement are detailed in the stages of motor development.

There are some important things to mention regarding stages of motor development. First is, although we rotate our heads in the early stages (baby #1) it is not a central theme of our movement, movement along the sagittal plane is. Sagittal plane movement is emphasized in the first three stages. Secondly, head rotation is thought to be more instinctive (searching for breast milk) rather than deliberate.

Every stage of motor development has a central theme and plane of movement and we've broken it down in the order described. Distinguishing movement in the planes can be easily confused and the labeling of the directions, from calling it movement along one plane then switching to calling it movement along another plane can be an exercise in fuzzy logic but we have to make sure we are describing a plane from the vertical axis since this is how we ended, in standing! This order of movement in the planes is called. This is the Order of Complexity.

The Order of Complexity

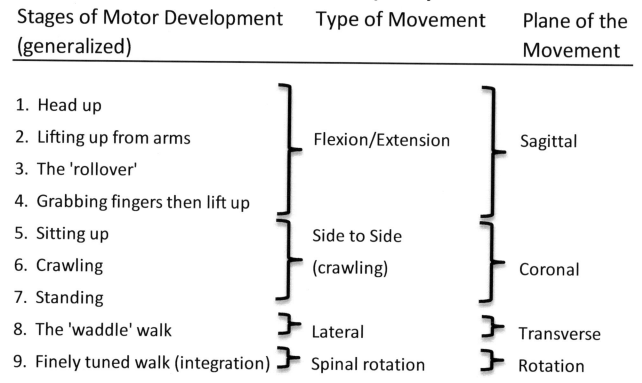

Stages of Motor Development (generalized)	Type of Movement	Plane of the Movement
1. Head up		
2. Lifting up from arms	Flexion/Extension	Sagittal
3. The 'rollover'		
4. Grabbing fingers then lift up		
5. Sitting up	Side to Side (crawling)	Coronal
6. Crawling		
7. Standing		
8. The 'waddle' walk	Lateral	Transverse
9. Finely tuned walk (integration)	Spinal rotation	Rotation

A Bit More on Transverse movement

When it comes to transverse movement, we have to make a distinction as to what it is. When doing visual assessments, we will isolate transverse movement to the areas that are capable of movement in the transverse planes and **can go into lateral movement, along the vertical axis**. The talus and the pelvis as a whole come to mind. When a client walks and they bend side to side in their walking we will describe that movement as happening along/in the coronal plane. Why is it not movement along the transverse plane? As noted before, we need to make a distinction here and we will say that walking with a side to side bend travels more along the coronal than in any other plane and so we will label it as movement along the coronal plane. Keeping this distinction of movement is very important because it will help us to break down all the information we're getting when we see a client walk, which can be a lot. Eventually it will also help us to determine a course of action when it comes to myo-fascial work because we may be able to add function in a particular plane of movement by working along the plane or promoting movement in the plane.

I tell my students that if they feel they can't see something the instructor is pointing out it may not be so much that they can't see it but it could be that they are seeing too much! I then offer the idea of breaking things down into planes. What's happening just in the sagittal plane, then the coronal plane, then the transverse plane and then finally in rotation. This way will help the practitioner to see things in a more pragmatic way and be less overwhelmed by what's happening in front of them.

NOTES

2 BODY READING

Before we proceed with the exercise of assessing the client it's important to understand that we ourselves can find it difficult to be objective in our readings. Emotionally, we need to be aware that we can empathize too much with the client or project thoughts and beliefs associated with their movement or posture. Physically, it's important to understand that we may be biased based on our judgment of what we believe to be 'proper' or what we believe looks 'good'. Being aware of where we're coming from or what we bring to the table so to speak will allow us to pull away from our own sense of self and understand where our clients are coming from.

This leads to a story. In the very beginning of my Rolfing practice I had a young lady come in to experience the ten series of sessions. She had complained about low back pain and wanted that to be the theme of the ten series. We were probably around session three or four when her low back pain had started to dissipate. As I got her to walk at the end of the session, I said, "wow, you're really walking like Marilyn Monroe!" thinking that was a compliment or at least an indication of progress. She instantly stopped walking and didn't say much afterwards. When she came back for her next session she complained of back pain again. I wasn't sure what, if anything, I did wrong but we had to back track and take care of the back issue. At the end of the session I noticed something when she got dressed. My client was dressed in a big flannel over-jacket, trousers, and tucked her hair into her cap. It was then I realized that by me saying that Marilyn Monroe comment I was interfering with her identity as a person and not taking into consideration how saying something like that could have an effect on her. From that point on I kept my comments neutral, saying how her pelvis seemed to be moving with more ease, and how she seemed to be able to move her pelvis in walking without experiencing pain. Over the subsequent sessions my client improved greatly and I learned a valuable lesson about being aware of and respecting all aspects of someone's identity. At the end of the series my client mentioned how she felt so good that she was going to take up salsa dancing with her partner! I said, "that's great!" and kept any possible references to Shakira to myself.

This is not a science, this is a craft.
We continue with the craft until science catches up

> **Is there a path that can lead a client to dysfunction? Yes. It's possible to think of this work in this way:**
> **1. Function exists 2. It can be influenced/affected by a habitual pattern, physical trauma, or psychological trauma 3. This can then lead to tissue dysfunction/pattern of dysfunction 4. The practitioner may be able to 'see' the dysfunction via body reading and palpate this dysfunction in the tissue as 'Directional Resistance'**

When starting the initial task of body reading it's important to understand that we can ask ourselves many questions about what may be going on with a client as they move and walk. We can attempt to determine everything that may be going on in one fell swoop but instead we need to be open to 'seeing' and working on the first few things that jump out at us. As my teachers have taught me, one of the biggest questions you will ask yourself as a practitioner of this craft is, "where do you go first"? Those first few things that jump out at us and that very first place we work on are the way that we as practitioners will work with and on our clients and how we approach them from an individual standpoint. This is one of the big things that makes this type of work stand out from all others.

I suggest you practice this type of body reading with a set of bodyworker friends. Take turns doing this exercise. Wear comfortable shorts that aren't too long and a sports bra if necessary. One at a time, have your colleague walk up and down in a straight line and as they're walking ask yourself the following questions about their body in movement. Please note that these are by far not the only questions to ask but they are a great place to start.

Dominant Eye

As you see someone walk and you attempt to assess them, understand that most of us have a dominant eye. If you have a dominant eye, let's say the left one for example, then if you're doing a walking assessment you might get different information standing on one side of the room than you would standing on the other. In order to maximize you're visual assessment, make sure you're seeing mostly from your dominant eye, if you have one. In order to determine which is your dominant eye, do this exercise: Stand relaxed and look at an object through an opening created by both your hands as they are making a triangle shape (your arms are outstretched). Make sure both eyes are open as you do this. Now close one eye. Is the object still visible? If so, then the open eye is your dominant eye. Switch the open and closed eyes. If the object disappears from your view then that confirms your dominant eye is not the eye you're currently using.

The Feet

When looking at the feet in walking, focus on a few areas at a time and ask yourself if you can determine an answer based on what you're seeing. Here are some of the things you would be looking for.

1. Is the toe hinge bending at all and supporting the client in walking? Is the toe hinge bend happening more on lateral toes rather than the medial toes or vice versa? A lack of toe hinge in

walking may indicate lack of movement in the ankle joint and tightness in the posterior part of the lower leg. It could also indicate a walking pattern left from an old injury.

2. How much time is the heel spending on the floor? Too much or not enough? If the answer is too much then that might indicate the client is shuffling their feet and maybe they don't have the ability to lengthen in the myo-fascial tissue in their legs and even their pelvis. Not enough time would look like they are bouncing up and down when they walk and that often results from tight lower leg tissue, especially the posterior lower leg.

3. When looking at the calcaneus, notice if it's supporting the talus in walking. Does the calcaneus move medially or laterally as the client takes their step and lands on that foot? If the calcaneus is not fully supporting the talus then we know there might be tight tissue either medially for a varus foot or laterally for a valgus foot.

4. When looking at the medial arch, ask yourself is it collapsing too much or completely flat in walking? Now try to imagine how a collapsing arch can affect toe hinge! Also look at the lateral arch, is it too tight such that it doesn't allow for proper push off of the foot? A tight lateral arch can make it so that the calcaneus shifts medially when walking and the heel 'slides in' as it hits the floor. If that's happening, the lateral arch needs to be assessed as it may be too tight.

5. Watching the talus in walking, specifically look at tibio-talar joint, see if it's moving well, meaning, is it articulating evenly in walking. The foot could be coming up prematurely because of inflexibility in the tibio-talar joint? There could also be foot valgus or varus due to uneven articulation in the tibio-talar joint. As extra food for thought, ask yourself how the tibio-talar joint could possibly affect (or get affected by) the hamstring area.

6. When looking at the navicular remember it moves inferiorly during walking, slightly moving inferiorly, then back up superiorly as the medial arch regains its form. Is the navicular moving too inferiorly during walking (this would happen when the arch collapses too much in walking) or is it not moving at all?

Knees

The knee is an interesting part of the body. It's strong yet mobile and often takes up the stress of tight areas above or below it. Because of this combination we tend to see knee issues and are quick to put the fault on this amazing joint when the structural integrity could be compromised from another part of the body.

1. In walking, during the heel strike phase, is the knee directly over the foot? Is it being supported by the foot?

2. If the knee is not directly overhead the foot, what would that mean for the tissue laterally and medially to the knee?

3. Look up the Screw-Home mechanism to understand what happens to the knee in walking. Is there a proper Screw-Home effect, adequate rotation of the femur and tibia in walking? If not, what tissue territories could be short/tight as a result?

A knee that is not supported by the foot and moves either medially or laterally in walking can mean that tissue in the adductor area is either too tight or weak or strained.

The Greater Trocanter

This area can be used as an indicator or marker for other things happening to the pelvis and in turn other parts of the body.

1. Looking at the greater trochanter: Is there proper circular movement with the trochanter in the

sagittal plane, in the shape of a "U". If we don't see that or if the trochanter moves in a different plane other than the sagittal plane, what territory may be preventing or 'hiding' this "U" movement? It could be that tightness in the gluteal area makes the trochanter move more laterally (along the transverse plane) than in the sagittal plane.

2. Is one trochanter moving more than the other or less than the other? This could indicate a tightness or restriction in the area where there is less movement and a hyper-mobility in the area where there is more movement.

One exercise we do in class is to walk with our classmates, behind them, with hands on the trochanters. As our classmates walks in a straight line, we feel how the trochanters move, either more in a superior/inferior manner, or in a more unilateral fashion, one side moving more laterally while the other trochanter barely moves at all for example. This example could also be indicative of sacro-iliac joint restrictions or unilateral tightness in the gluteal muscles.

Quadriceps and Hamstrings

There are many different ways to look at this area of the leg. In this case we will look at how they interact with the adductors and how they move along the rotational axis.

1. Looking at quads and hamstrings in walking, how are they moving or 'rolling' on the femur. This may not be clearly evident at first so we can ask ourselves instead, are the adductors presenting themselves more in the anterior leg or the posterior leg when our client walks towards us and away from us? Anterior presentation means they are moving more with the quadriceps and thus the quadriceps are rolling more laterally along the femur. Posterior presentation of the adductors in walking may indicate that the adductors are moving more with the hamstrings and thus the quadriceps are moving more medially when walking and the hamstrings are also moving more laterally.

Psoas and Trunk

The psoas muscle territory can be seen as an extension of the leg. Functionally, it helps the leg move and aids in hip flexion. When there is no functional connection/awareness in the client between leg and psoas, then the client may walk showing a distinct separation between the lower half and the upper half of their body. We see this with people who sit a lot for a living like delivery drivers.

> **In this type of work we look at the psoas muscle as an extension of the leg, which we can call the 'functional leg'**

1. In walking, where does the leg functionally end (in the superior part)? A leg that doesn't resonate its movement in the psoas area may end up using additional energy for locomotion and exhibiting movement from other parts of the body, such as the quadriceps.

2. Looking at pelvis/trunk area: Is it moving only along the transverse plane or only along the sagittal plane (or maybe even coronal)? Does it look like the muscles of the pelvis are keeping it from moving? Does it look like the muscles may be overworking because other areas are not working as much?

3. Does it look like the pelvic bowl is 'sucked into' the body? This can be indicated by the client's

clothing (their shorts) getting 'sucked up' into their pelvic floor.

4. Pelvic Tilt/Shift: In standing and in walking, where is the pelvis in relation to the rest of the body? Does the pelvis move before everything else or is it the last part to move? This would point more towards pelvic shift. In looking for tilt, is the ASIS (anterior superior iliac spine) pointing more inferiorly as the whole pelvis tilts forward (this would happen with an anterior tilt) or is the opposite happening, which would indicate a posterior tilt. Ask yourself how would that affect the client's walk.

Torso and Spine

In this initial body reading, we start to examine the rest of the core and how it behaves and interacts with itself and other parts of the body.

1. Looking at the torso we want to understand how the chest and abs allow the client to move forward in space. Are the abs tight to the extent that they keep the client's torso in a flexed position? Do the abdominals seem to pull down on the pectoralis area when walking?

2. Are there any rotational patterns or adhesions between the abdominals and the chest, meaning do the abdominals rotate more in one direction than the other when the client performs contralateral movement in walking?

3. Keep in mind this body reading analysis only covers the surface. More exploration can be done that examines the viscera, the lungs and diaphragm.

4. Looking at the back: Is the Structural Vertical Axis (or, what we may call core) aligning itself with the Functional Vertical Axis (or, where the client rotates from when walking. Keep in mind that the functional vertical axis is that area where the client rotates along and this area may differ from the structural axis, or midline. A difference in the Structural and Functional Vertical Axis is evident when you see a client walking in such a way that one side of their body rotates medially more so than the other but away from the central axis. The body reader may pick it up as seeing more movement on one side that the other.

5. Looking at the spine should include a study of Serge Gracovetsky and Gracovetsky's Chains of Movement. This will show us that the spine moves in a rotational pattern during contra-lateral movement. Ideally, we want to see this type of movement all along the spine in our clients. When we see our client walk, is there an area of the spine that is 'still' and not moving as much and could use more movement? Check out Youtube for videos on Gracovetsky and his research.

Some food for thought: When looking at the back with the client in walking keep in mind that if the right foot is turned out (externally rotated), then that could prompt the right side of the back to activate more than usual during contra-lateral movement. When the right foot and leg are straight on and move along the sagittal plane, then the left side (contra-lateral) 'turns on' or activates more. Lengthening the right side may promote proper contra-lateral movement. Lengthening may start with the foot.

Shoulder Girdle, Forearm, and Hand

1. Looking at the Gleno-humeral joint: Does the humerus seem to move at ease in the socket joint when the arm swings in walking? Does the humerus move along the sagittal plane or does it cross the plane? Does it move at all? Is it turned medially or laterally? If it turns medially, is this internal rotation happening at the humerus or somewhere else?

2. In static, is one scapula more 'winged' out than the other (possible weakness and/or tightness (long and tight) in the serratus anterior area.

3. In walking, do the scapulae stay still/motionless or is there movement? Is there too much movement from the whole shoulder girdle? Too much movement could be a compensation for not much movement in the pelvic area. Check the pelvic area for lack of movement.

4. Does the shoulder girdle hang from the neck or does it settle over the ribcage? Basically, what area is the shoulder girdle 'belonging' to? What we are looking for here is restriction and where the restriction is most related to, an upper portion or lower portion.

5. Looking at the forearm and hand: Is the forearm supinated or pronated when walking? Do we see the palm of the hand more or the back of the hand? Ideally, we are looking for a more neutral position.

An arm that crosses the sagittal plane when the client is walking could be indicative of tightness in the pectoralis area (including but not limited to brachioradialis) and overly stretched/possibly weak tissue in the infraspinatus area.

Head and eyes

The head and eyes can direct the rest of the body. Affecting this top part of the core affects the rest of the body. In a lot of martial arts, especially the grappling arts, it's often taught that the body will follow where the head is pointing and directed so direction your opponent's head is key. Emphasis is given on being able to control the head to control the whole person. In body reading we can look at how the client uses their head and ask ourselves:

1. Is the head down or up in walking? Where is the person's gaze when they walk? Is the head tilted to one side? Does the head bob up or down? Is the head forward or backward in walking?

Many times when a client knows they are being watched and assessed they will often feel judged and will adjust their gait to make the practitioner feel good or to walk in the way they feel they 'should' walk.

A few things I do to help with this is to have the client walk and stop and see what the difference is from the beginning of their walk and the end of it. I sometimes look away when the client is looking towards me and look at them when they are looking away in order to get a more relaxed gait from the client. When the client starts to walk again I quickly look at their gaze. Where did they gaze fall when they started walking? Did they look down as they started to walk or did they look up?

Other Body Reading Models - The G/G' Model

As we have seen from our previous body reading questions, we are looking at the body from a perspective of articulation along different planes. This is just one way of reading and assessing people. There is another model that is also an interesting perspective and it's called the G/G' model.

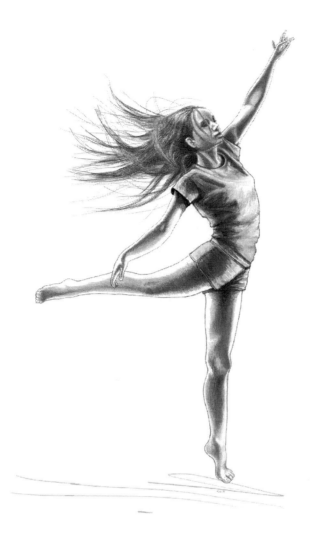

The G/G' model (as taught to me by Monica Caspari) assumes that people are predisposed to either be more upper body **(G' being around T3)** or lower body **(G being typically in the pelvis)** gravity oriented. G refers to the lower body center of gravity orientation and G' refers to the upper body orientation. When someone is more oriented towards a lower center of gravity oriented for example, different compensation patterns and areas of tightness can arise. A simple way to see if your client leans towards G or G' is to have them start and stop walking. When they start up again, look at how they use their body to start the motion. Do they slightly flex forward (at their trunk) or does their sternum seem to move superiorly as they take their first step? A G oriented person may sink a tiny bit towards the floor and/or flex forward as they take their first step. A G' oriented person may seem to float up towards the ceiling as they taking their first step. Ask yourself, are you more G or G' oriented?

Going on to Youtube you can watch videos with Fred Astaire and Gene Kelly dancing together. They were both masters of their art but both come at it from different orientations. One is more G oriented while the other is a classic G'. After watching a video can you see which one is which?

Now that we have a sense of what we're looking for, we can assess the related muscle tissue and apply certain goals to our work. Overall, we can make it a goal to balance tissue and give our client more ease in movement.

A great way to get a sense of what may be happening in your client is to mimic their walking. This is different than mocking your client. Try to do it as they are walking and walk behind them. This will give you a sense of how they bring movement and what areas in their body may be tight/short. You may have noticed that this chapter was full of a lot of questions without a whole lot of answers. Some of the questions asked can be answered by mimicking the client's walk. The body comes with so many answers already built in and a lot of times all that is needed is to listen.

3 TERRITORY ASSESSMENT

Now that we have visually assessed and have an idea of what may be going on, the next step is to confirm what we see with palpation. Assessment through palpation is not just a matter of touching the tissue. If we visually assess and we determine some possible anomaly in function, what do we expect to find in the tissue? What we do is feel for Directional Resistance. What is that? Finding Directional Resistance comes from first understanding that tissue (myo-fascial tissue) can be directionally resistant, regardless of the direction of the muscle fibers. This means that myo-fascial tissue will feel like it can move more easily in one direction versus another. Directional Resistance can occur due to a habitual pattern that will leave some myo-fascial areas of the body shorter and tighter than others. Directional Resistance can occur anywhere in the body and transcends muscles or muscle groups.

> **SI Visual Assessment + Specific Palpation Assessment (Directional Resistance/Ease) + Specific Myo-fascial Bodywork + Principles/Rules of SI = Structural Integration approach**

In order to buy into this model you have to accept that tension does not only exist at an attachment or at a bony protuberance. Tension can exist anywhere when we think myo-fascial (fascia after all, doesn't have a specific origin or insertion).

To take it a step further, Directional Resistance (dr) can vary from location to location in a particular muscle and can vary from layer to layer in a muscle group or individual muscle. This is because the muscle cell could be influenced in direction by the collagen fibers surrounding it. This means that dr could be influenced by the state of the muscle cell and also by the state of the fascia and connective tissue; Directional Resistance is myo-fascial or put in a more general term: myo-connective tissue. Going forward, the terms myo-fascial and myo-connective tissue may be used interchangeably.

Working to add more length/fluidity/release/etc. in the direction that the tissue is resistant is a very direct method of work and thus this type of myo-fascial bodywork is called a Direct Method. Other types of work that don't work this way could be classified under Indirect Method. So, the next step in assessment would be to marry the two assessment techniques (visual and palpation) into a way of assessment. This entails first the visual assessment and then the confirmation of the visual findings by seeing if the dr matches our visual findings. This way adds to specificity and may lead to quicker results. Let's take the example of fallen arches.

Fallen arches are a very common scenario and its effects can be seen all throughout the leg and body.

Let's imagine the chain of events that can happen (these are just possibilities) by this when someone with fallen arches is walking and we will use the visual assessment questions we asked ourselves earlier to help us pinpoint certain areas of their body that might be moving in a dysfunctional pattern:

1. Navicular 'meets' the floor at an extreme level, doesn't 'rise' back up, possibly causing the foot to externally rotate
2. Talus shifts medially in the heel strike phase of the step
3. Tibio-Talar joints bends non-horizontally (possibly more bend at the lateral part than the medial part)
4. Tibia rotates internally more than externally when observing the Screw-Home effect
5. Knee and Femur moves medially, knee is not directly over the foot when the foot lands and thus the knee is not supported by the foot
6. Greater trochanter rotates internally
7. Corresponding Ilium inflares

In addition to these boney territories, the myo-fascial tissue could be short/tight in these areas:

1. Lateral arch tissue
2. Lateral retinaculum
3. Tissue around Tibia/Fibula rotated internally
4. Strain in Pes Anserinus
5. IT Band tightness
6. Short and tight in Superior Adductors/Pelvic bowl
7. Tightness in TFL/upper Lateral Rotators, lower lateral rotators could be short
8. Shortness in Iliacus area
9. Gluteus maximus could be tight/taut on the superior part of the tissue
10. Deeper glutes (the lateral rotators) could be long and taut on the superior part and short and tight for the lower lateral rotator territory
11. Adductors could be long and taut
12. Pubic bone could have a tendency to shift medially
13. The psoas at the lesser trochanter could be rotated medially

Now let's imagine possible Directional Resistance outcomes for this same situation:

1. Lateral arch tissue is tight and could have dr in the distal direction, meaning it may be more resistant upon palpation for the tissue to go distally, towards the toes, than towards the heel
2. Tissue around Tibia/Fibula rotated internally and could therefore be more resistant in the external direction
3. IT Band tightnesss and possible dr in the superior/proximal direction, especially by the knee joint
4. Tightness in TFL/upper Lateral Rotators and possible dr going from anterior to posterior
5. Shortness in Iliacus area and possible dr going from inferior to superior

Can you imagine those possibilities? The following are some graphical representations of Directional Resistance.

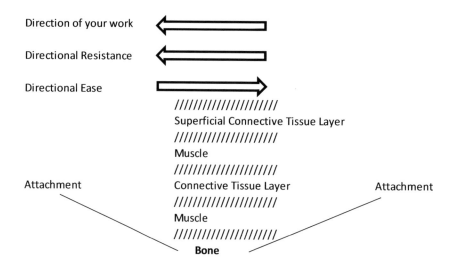

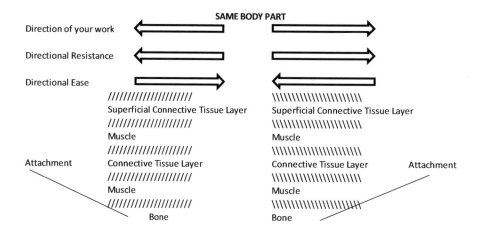

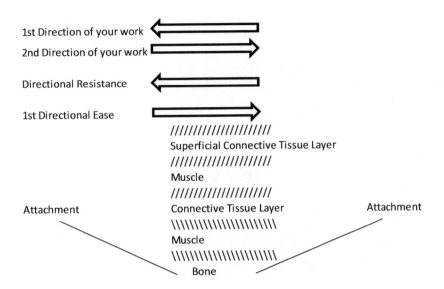

Now let's cover some territories that we would palpate after a visual assessment. These are not all the areas but just an overview in order to understand the concept of palpatory assessment. Feel free to create your own repertoire keeping in mind that we are confirming our visual assessment and checking for Directional Resistance in order to create a game plan for future work. Since this is a system of work, we seek to connect what we see with our palpation assessment and relate that information to the client's possible dysfunctions. With practice, it's possible to see the relationships.

Tibio-Talar Joint area

1. Palpate the talus and check for ease in dorsiflexion and plantar flexion. Approximately 20 degrees of dorsiflexion is necessary in running for example.
2. Feel for the navicular and which way it wants to move more naturally, either superiorly or inferiorly.
3. Check for tightness in tendon/ligament tissue around navicular.
4. Check for foot valgus or varus. A foot varus in the ankle joint will have tight tissue in the medial ankle and may have dr going in the inferior direction.
5. Feel for tightness in lateral arch and ease of movement in cuboid bone.

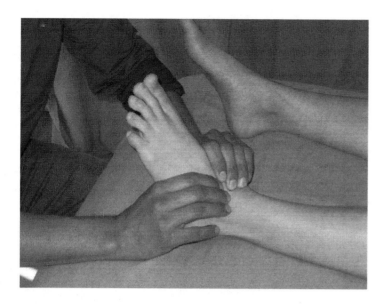

Knees

1. Perform knee sleeve work. Hold both hands on the top of the knee, around the patella and more your hands in opposing directions (for example, your right hand rotating internally while your left hand, which is superior to the patella, rotates externally). and feel for which direction is more restricted. Then switch your direction with each hand. Feel again for directional resistance.

2. Perform 'knee sleeve' work with both hands moving in the superior/inferior direction; one hand moving superiorly while the other moves inferiorly. Switch directions of your hands so that your hands are now moving to the same central point, the patella (without of course putting direct pressure on the patella).

3. Palpate the proximal and distal areas of the fibula and feel for ease of movement. When we walk we have movement in the fibula but the fibula doesn't take on as much weight as the tibia so keep that in mind. Check for balance between both fibulas. If you found one leg that had less lower leg movement (maybe there wasn't enough Screw-Home mechanism) than the other, then how does that relate to the movement of the fibula in palpation?

Note that in the previous scenario with the fallen arches, it's possible that the hand on the superior part of the patella would have trouble rotating externally and moving superiorly.

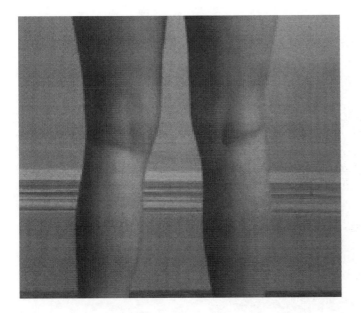

Knees (continued)

1. Look at back of knees and where the hamstrings attach, which hamstrings could be pulling more on the back of knee tissue? If the lateral hamstrings seem to be pulling more on the back of the knee you might also see the horizontal crease in the back of the knee angle more in the superior direction on the lateral side. The dr of the tissue on the lateral side could be inferiorly (meaning, the tissue is more resistant going in the inferior direction, from somewhere in the mid/lower hamstring area to the back of the knee.

Greater Trocanter

1. Palpate the tissue around the greater trocanter (with your client in sidelying position) and see which way it wants to go and which way it doesn't want to go (directional resistance). Identify the tissue that is in the area that is more restricted. This creates a gameplan for future work.

Pelvis/Sacrum

1. In standing, have client flex forward (reaching for toes). Check to see which side of the sacrum is restricted (this is the one that moves first and moves superiorly). With client in prone, palpate the ilium, in the PSIS area, looking for which side doesn't have as much 'bounce'. The less 'bouncy' area may have tighter glute tissue and tighter tissue around the sacrum. Check then for Directional Resistance.

2. Feel for dr in the gluteal muscles along the sagittal and coronal planes. Do the restrictions correlate to what was seen with the client walking?

Spinal Column

1. When assessing the spinal column along the sagittal plane, one way to do this is to have the client on their side. Palpating about an inch and a half from the spinous process 'bounce' on the tissue, meaning feel for range of motion of a particular vertebra by taking it in the anterior/posterior direction. Usually this is done with a finger or thumb on either side from the spine. If there is tightness then this might indicate lack of mobility in that particular area.

2. Feel for tightness in the erector/fascial layer with your open
palm, using your full hand including fingers. Without pressing down on the spinous processes, use one or both hands to move tissue clockwise and counter-clockwise, on either side of the spinal column, noticing which area doesn't move as easy and which direction doesn't move as easily. In this case we are working with superficial fascia, not with multifidus or rotatores tissue and we are assessing in the coronal plane.

Gleno-Humeral Joint
1. Holding the Gleno-humeral joint firmly, feel for where it wants to move and where it doesn't. Hold the posterior part of the joint and feel for how the rotator cuff muscles allow or don't allow the humerus to rotate. In the photo, I am holding the clavicle and scapula firmly with my right hand while my left hand moves the humerus anteriorly and posteriorly and then in internal and external rotation. These moves are done slowly and methodically, never with any type of thrust or undue force. We are basically looking to see if the restrictions (if any) in this area are due to joint restrictions or due to tight tissue restrictions.

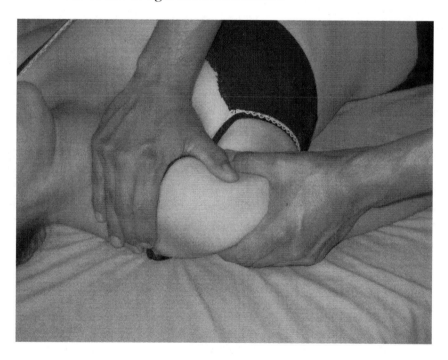

Pectoralis Major
1. Feel the tissue of the pectoralis major and notice, which direction does it want to move? Medially rotated arms could have pectoralis major tissue that is directionally resistant in the lateral/superior direction for example.

Scapula and related myo-fascia
1. With your client in prone, rotate the scapula clockwise and counter-clockwise and notice which is easier to do. Which myo-connective tissue may be restricting the movement of the scapula? For example if you are holding the client's right scapula in your left hand and you rotate the scapula clockwise, and you notice restriction, the tissue in the teres major/teres minor territory could be

restricting scapular movement. Keep in mind that the serratus anterior muscle could also be restrictive but only in certain parts of that muscle (serratus anterior inferior). The serratus anterior could also be tight and weak in certain parts.

Lower Arm and Hand
1. With client in supine, feel for which way the arm naturally wants to rest.
2. Feel for which way it more comfortably wants to turn, in supination or in pronation?
3. Palpate the wrists and notice which way is easier for the wrist to move, flexion or extension?
4. Feel the muscles/connective tissue of the thenar eminence and

flexors of the hand, are they tight? Is the hand in constant flexion? What is the Directional Resistance of the thenar eminence tissue?

Head and Neck
1. In supine, palpate the sterno-cleidomastoid muscles. Which way does the muscle like to move, in external rotation or internal rotation. Is it easy for that muscle to separate itself from the cervical myo-fascia underneath it?
2. Run your fingers along the cervical spine, making stripes on the posterior neck muscles, determine how tight the upper trapezius muscles are and what areas may need work. Feel for ease of movement in their neck, in lateral flexion and rotation. Checking for lateral flexion means making sure there is movement along the sagittal plane.
3. Focus on particular parts of the client's neck and check for movement along the coronal plane by side-bending gently along each vertebra. Does a possible restriction match what was see in walking?
4. For the head, feel the scalp and while holding the skull securely by the occiput, feel for restrictions and dr in the scalp. If a client tilts their head to their right when walking for example, do you experience dr towards their left when assessing? Care must be taken to not compress the client's neck which is why a firm hold should be performed by their occiput.

One thing that's very important to understand is that the palpation of the tissue from the territory in question is also palpated while keeping the plane in mind . We are not palpating randomly or palpating just in order to start working on whatever we feel is tight. Instead, we may feel for dr in one plane and then another plane and then from there we can make the decision to work in and along the planes based on the Order of Complexity. Assessing the territory via palpation will help us to determine a cause of action with performing manual therapy. For example, if we can check for ease of movement in flexion/extension, then for ease in side-bending (along the coronal plane) we are keeping the planes in mind.

A quick palpation of the skull can also include keeping the planes in mind. Moving the skull tissue in the planes from the Order of Complexity will reveal some interesting correlations with the skull tissue and tissue and territories in the body.

4 MYO-FASCIAL TECHNIQUES

With Morales Method® Core Integration, we aim to work myo-fascial tissue (in addition to other tissue such as nerve and visceral tissue) but it's important to understand fascia to get a big picture sense of what is happening under our hands. Fascia is the connective tissue that is completely continuous, and holds us together, it's been described as the 'organ of support'. It is made up of a web of collagen fibers (proteins) that hold and support many important structures and it also reacts to our bodywork/mechanical pressure. In this type of work we work with, among other tissue, superficial fascia that travels through the body like planes and also with areas where fascia gets thicker and 'dives' into the body, creating a thick line of tissue, or septum. **We are also aware and work with areas that may not necessarily have a name but still register under our palpation as tight areas of connective tissue that display Directional Resistance**. It's important to note that these levels/planes that we imagine in our minds exist only in our minds, the myo-fascial system in our bodies does not distinguish between levels or planes, it is a construct that we have created in order to create a strategy/approach.

We start to understand through this type of work by realizing that one area of the body can affect other areas. We begin to see that with visual assessment. We then confirm this relationship by working the tissue in a certain way and in certain directions (this is determined when we do a palpation assessment). We then start to understand that working one area of the body will affect another area. This is the beginning of understanding Structural Integration. Once we understand the philosophy of Structural Integration and start to incorporate certain rules, our work starts to become Structural Integration.

In working different areas of the body we will follow different philosophies and ways of thinking. For example, we often work superficial fascia before we work deeper layers of fascia (this is covered in more detail in the upcoming chapters). In the Morales Method® We strive not to follow one form or get tied to just one protocol but move within trains of thought to 'get the job done'.

Structural Integration is a thinking person's game. In the beginning a protocol is introduced to the practitioner for them to follow. Following this protocol is meant to help the practitioner get familiar with working myo-fascia in a specific way and to start to see the body from a Structural Integration perspective. It is when we start to understand the body from this perspective that we can comfortably let go of the protocol and start to 'play jazz'. Attempting to do Structural Integration without learning a protocol is the equivalent of breaking a rule without truly knowing or understanding the rule in the first place. The work then takes on a haphazard form.

The following techniques are only to be used if necessary. Every single one of the following techniques are not meant to be done on the client every single time. Also, these are not the only techniques that can be used, there are many others, these are just a highlight of the many different ways to work the myo-fascia with a client. As you learn more about Structural Integration you are expected to learn them, practice them and utilize them when you feel the need to. Sit up, crawl, stand, walk, and then dance, just like we did when we were babies!

Keep in mind the properties of the connective tissue you're working with. Connective tissue, in this case myo-fascial tissue, is made up of muscle tissue and collagen fibers which are proteins. These collagen proteins are hydrophilic, are thought to have a piezoelctric effect, and can create 'gluey burrs' between layers, what we may classically feel as adhesions.

For more information on fascia read the book, "Fascia: The Tensional Network of the Human Body" by Robert Schleip

---

When working myo-fascial tissue we will be working with different philosophies in mind. Although not covered in great detail at this point, they are part of the way we work in Structural Integration. Some terms to keep in mind are: Working in planes, working along planes, directional resistance, and directional ease.

When going through the visual assessment exercises what we were actually doing was looking at how the body articulates at certain points and how it moves along and through certain planes. What we were also doing was creating a strategy for future work. Jan Sultan, a world renowned Rolfing® instructor once told the class I was in that as bodyworkers we were going to ask ourselves three main questions throughout our career:

1. Where do I go to first?
2. Where do I go to next?
3. How and when do I exit/close this session?

These words have carried me through a successful career and have inspired me to think deeply about how I work with my clients. As a Structural Integrator you are far from haphazardly working with tissue in all directions for the mere sake of massaging the tissue. You are always thinking about what is happening under your hands and what is happening to your client as a result.

The model for body reading can be described as the

MOVEMENT in PLANES/ARTICULATION model

The other point I want to make is that as we are working myo-fascia, we want to make sure we are taking tissue (for the purposed of using the Direct Method) in the direction it is most resistant and also taking the tissue to its end range. If you do not take the tissue to its end range you are not facilitating the fluidity in the tissue necessary to spark a possible change. The following photos will show techniques I use every day. Keep in mind that the direction of your work will change based on what you feel the Directional Resistance is, so your technique may vary. Although with most of this work we may end up going in the direction of resistance it may also be necessary to go with the tissue in the direction of ease. This type of work is better known as Positional Release and I've found it to be a great complement to this work.

A Brief Guideline to Myo-Fascial Techniques

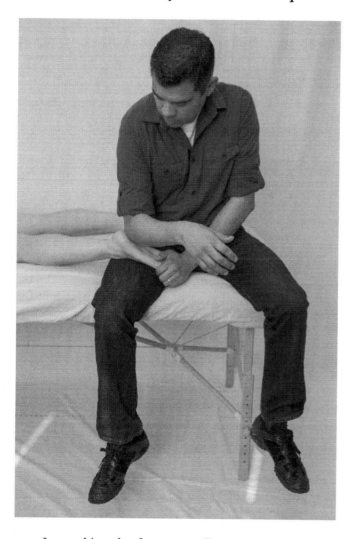

In working the foot, we will attempt to bring articulation to the areas we saw as 'stuck' or 'still' from our previous visual assessment. If I noticed that my client was shuffling their feet in walking, I may work the posterior leg area, check for proper tibio-talar movement, and also work the plantar part of the foot, in this case working the plantar fascia.

Plantar fascia: Work in this area can done using both thumbs to work from outside to inside. Imagine 'slicing' or 'filleting' the tissue in order to stretch and relieve tightness. Depending on dr, you could move either superiorly or inferiorly.

Talus: Encourage dorsiflexion by moving the foot into dorsi and plantar flexion, while keeping fingers in the tibio-talar joint, almost creating a wedge in that area. Keep in mind from your visual assessment that not the whole stretch of that joint needs to be working uniformly, the medial part of the tibio-talar joint may need more work than that lateral part of the joint if the client walked around with a laterally rotated foot or if their arch was collapsing in walking. This work can have profound effects on the rest of the client's body. Also, this can also be done in standing as seen in the photo. With the client in standing, my first and second toes are wedge into the tibio-talar portion that needs work and I ask my client to do a slow knee bend while keeping my toes in place. This technique uses their body weight to open up the restriction portion of the joint.

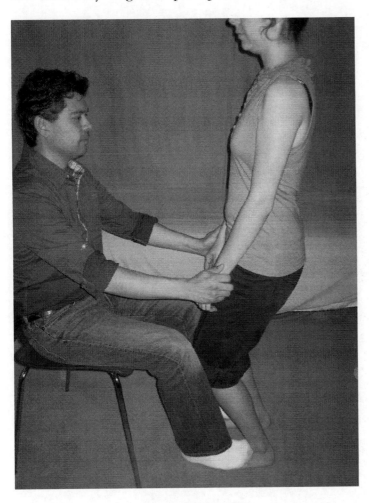

Malleoli area: This area will need work if the client is exhibiting foot valgus or varus. If the client has a foot varus, feel for tightness and dr in the medial malleolus. If the client exhibits foot valgus, feel for tightness and work in the direction of resistance in the lateral malleolus accordingly. In the classic Structural Integration philosophy working the feet is seen as a way to make sure the rest of your work has a strong basis for support. The feet work is seen as supporting future work. In MMCI, working the foot can add support future work but the feet can also be seen as reflecting issues happening above it (the pelvis area) hence, the feet are not always the first place to work.

Since the feet can be seen as an extension of the spine, (look at your embryological studies to see where the feet develop from) in MMCI we see the feet either supporting future work or reflecting bodywork performed in other territories. Either way, working the feet can mean bringing precise and particular mobility to all necessary parts of the foot. The study of embryology (embryo at three weeks) can inform your work.

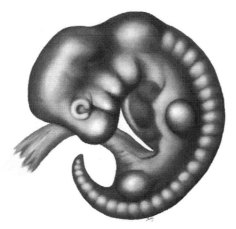

Embryo at three weeks

In MMCI we have a saying, "The feet are the spine". Looking at an image of an embryo at about three weeks, you can see the nubs of the legs and feet starting to develop from the area that will eventually become pelvis.

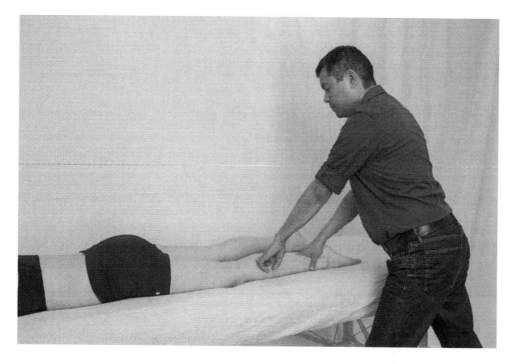

Lower leg: In prone, work the compartment holding the gastrocnemius and soleus. Move and differentiate that compartment with broad hands (in my workshops I call it using 'bear paws') to do superficial work. In a client with Plantar Fasciitis you might notice the tissue is more resistant going in the inferior direction. Palpate and work the septums in the areas where you feel dr. For example, working behind the fibula will allow you to access the Posterior Intermuscular Septum. If you have a client with Plantar Fasciitis, portions of this and other septums may also be resistant in the inferior direction which would mean you would work going inferiorly for that particular territory. Also, don't forget you can work the lower leg in sidelying position, working medial or lateral tissue. Make sure you understand where all the compartments of the lower leg are as these are areas where tightness can be housed. A hot bed of myo-fascial tightness are the anterior and posterior intermuscular septums.

Another area that comes to mind when working the lower leg is the area between the malleoli, in particular the deep part, connected by the inter-osseous membrane. This area, when tight and restricted, can limit the amount of dorsiflexion in the foot. One way I work it is hold the tibia and fibular head on the proximal part while moving/slowly twisting the malleoli on the distal end.

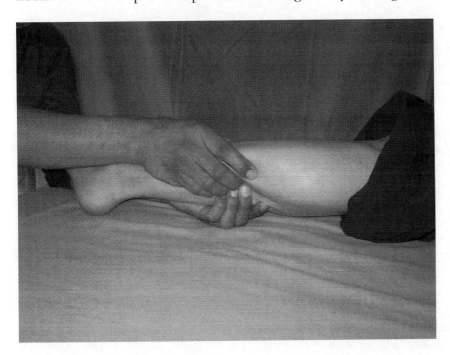

Sometimes I find myself having to work the lower leg with the client in supine position. From this underneath position, I can grip the area(s) that needs work and slowly lean back (if I need to go in the inferior direction) and work the myo-fascia that way. I can also imagine I am bringing separation to the different compartments in this location (this area is called the Superficial Posterior Compartment).

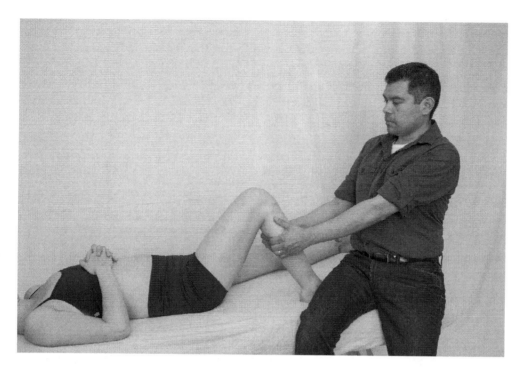

At this point I have only mentioned techniques that go along the sagittal plane. When we did a visual assessment we looked at the Screw-Home effect and how the lower leg moved internally and externally during walking. If you noticed and verified (through palpation) that the client's left lower leg for example moved more in internal rotation than the other, then we also need to work with the lower leg in the rotational direction. One way to work it would be to grip ('bear paw' again) and move the lower leg in the direction it's most resistant. A good overall grip is necessary here. Also, make sure you not putting undue torque on the knee joint, this is more of a myo-fascial technique.

Knees: This area is a fun yet complex area to work with. I often feel I don't do it justice when talking about it in a workshop and I feel that writing about it briefly would also not do it justice. Because of this I recommend Art Rigg's book, "Deep Tissue Massage" for a great primer on working the legs and knees. Besides this great resource, I recommend we use the 'knee sleeve' assessment technique as a way to work the knees. I usually take the tissue to its end range and hold it there, waiting for the tissue to become more fluid. Other areas to focus on are: Pes Anserinus, Patellar ligament, and the ilio-tibial band area by the tibia. All of these areas are worked keeping Directional Resistance in mind.

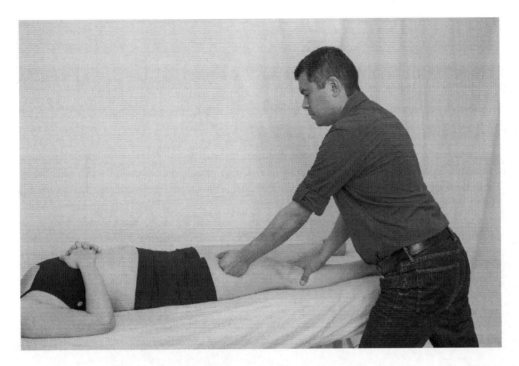

Quadriceps: A move made famous by Art Riggs is a superficial 'grab and move' technique. This move is initially intended to assess but can quickly become a therapeutic technique, much like the 'knee sleeve' work. 'Grab and move' the quadriceps as a whole to palpate which direction is most resistant. From there you can go to more detailed work by finding the areas and septums that are tight and their directional resistance. Use fingers, knuckles or a soft fist (as shown) to work the territory in the direction needed.

One interesting thing to note is the relationship between foot in dorsiflexion and the quadriceps. In some clients, when the foot is dorsiflexed (passively, by the practitioner) the quadriceps and leg may rotate internally. This may be due to unilateral tightness in the back of the leg (hamstrings and gastrocnemius muscles) that create an asymmetric pull on the leg. Working the quadriceps muscles in a rotational manner is key to bring symmetry to the leg but work needs to be done in posterior leg (behind the knee) in order to complete the work.

Other additional techniques I employ on the quadriceps include bringing separation between quads and adductors and on the lateral side bringing differentiation between quadriceps and the ilio-tibial band. This last technique is very effective in side-lying position.

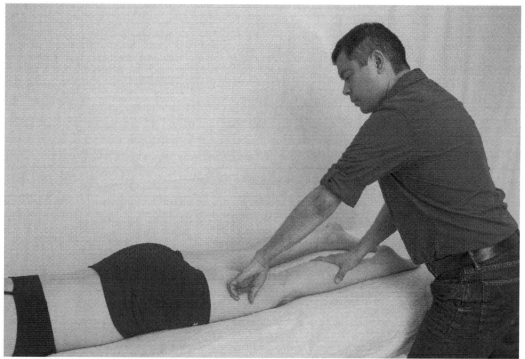

Hamstrings: Tightness in the hamstrings and lower leg will produce different fascial strains behind the knee that are visible as 'un-horizontal' lines as we saw from our visual assessment. Check for these lines in standing and in movement and work accordingly to make those lines more horizontal. For example, if we see our client with a lower leg that turns out (in walking or running) such that their foot 'kicks out' in their gait, a 'culprit' could be a tight lateral hamstring and the Directional Resistance could be in the inferior direction (meaning you would work going in the inferior direction). A practitioner of Structural Integration may also look at the relationship of the adductors in a person with this type of gait and see what would be going on in the pectineus area (possible shortness for example).

> Get familiar with palpating this area and know where all the attachments
> are, including the attachments for the popliteus and the plantaris. Also,
> know where the artery and nerve in that area run in order to avoid them.

I have often found that tightness in the distal hamstrings is accompanied by tightness in proximal lower leg and this naturally goes to working the back of the knee. Knowing how to work the back of the knee is important for the Structural Integration practitioner. As usual, feel for Directional Resistance of the tissue you aim to work and proceed.

Hamstrings: Work the fascial lines medial to the semitendinosus and lateral to the biceps femoris. This septum area can get tight, especially with runners and cyclists. Work in between the three hamstring muscles, feeling with fingers the fascial tissue that separates the individual hamstring muscles. You can imagine you are 'slicing' through the fascial line and you can move side to side, still keeping the septum under your fingers but moving the individual muscle from the fixed point of the septum. When you do this you may realize that you're working on rotation and although the hamstring muscles don't necessarily have rotation as an action, asymmetrical tightness of the hamstring muscles can cause internal or external rotation of the femur.

Also remember that the sacro-tuberus ligament represents a fascial extension of the hamstrings that go beyond the ischial tuberosity. Don't forget, work superficially before going deep (as in, doing sleeve work on the posterior knee) before diving into that area.

Hamstrings and quads can form a 'sticky' relationship with the adductors. Remember your assessment findings to know how to work on adductors and what position to best put your client in.

For more information on the latest research on fascia I suggest looking at the work of Robert Schleip and the research site: http://www.fasciaresearch.de

---

I am constantly in awe of the myo-connective tissue system we reside in. We are still in the beginning stages of learning of fascia and I'm grateful for being around at this time where so much is being learned about the work we do. Recently, we have found that fascia is dynamic, has contractile properties, and is 'hydrophilic', meaning it will take on fluid when interacted with.

Ida Rolf said, "As the pelvic floor gains support and balance, the tone of the whole viscera improves".

Obturator: During assessment, you may have noticed if the pelvic floor was too 'sucked into' the pelvis or if the pelvic floor seemed tight. Working the obturator is key in offering more span to the pelvic floor and good base of support for the rest of the body. If the pelvic floor is too tight, the legs may not move directly underneath the pelvis and the person may end up walking with an adaptation (pelvis moving transversely on one side for example). When working this territory you may notice its relationship to the adductor and inner line of the leg and above it, to the abdominal core.

Gluteal muscles: This territory can be worked in prone or in side-lying position. We can also begin working on a superficial level before diving in to deeper gluteal tissue. Use your deep tissue skills to work on deep lateral rotators, especially piriformis. Remember, piriformis affects sacral torsion and nutation. Any work in the deeper gluteal muscles should also follow the same method of working in between the septums of the muscles tissue, especially the piriformis.

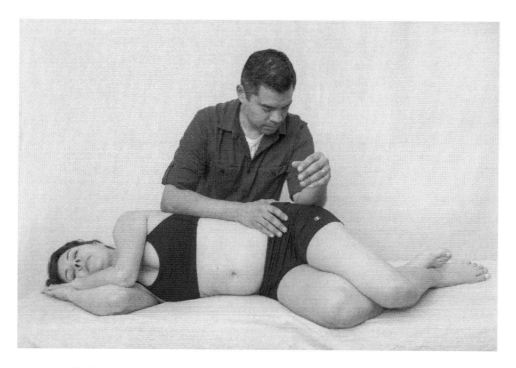

In side-lying, superficial work can look like this: rotate gluteal tissue clockwise and counter-clockwise using the greater trochanter as the center and feel for which area the gluteal tissue is more restricted. First work superficially moving surface tissue (gluteus maximus) in the direction it doesn't want to go. Then, use a forearm, fingers, or soft fist to still work the superficial myo-fasical layer of the gluteals. This work tends to focus on the sagittal plane and will help to bring more balance to a client who isn't walking as much in that plane (as previously discussed, someone whose pelvis is moving more transversely on one side).

When working the sacrum, use your tool of choice (fingers, knuckles, etc.) to work the fascia on top of the sacrum and along the ilium, working superficially, then deep. Your goal will be to 'free the sacrum' so to speak. I have noticed that a flat low back can be helped by working the sacrum area.

Now that we've ventured into side-lying work, it's important to bring up how to work this area keeping myo-fascia in mind. With my client in side-lying, I use both hands to move the fascia anterior to posterior. I can work inferior to superior or the other way around as well. I may often incorporate movement in this technique (asking the client to move/raise their arm as I work superior to inferior).

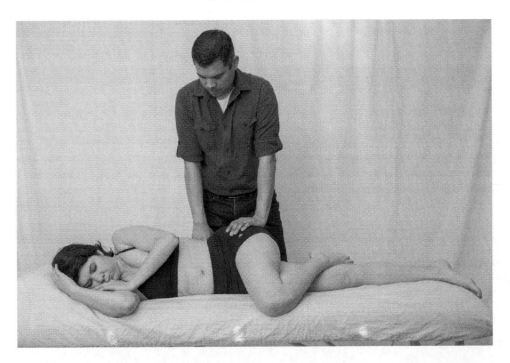

Erector Spinae: With the erectors, imagine 'slicing' or 'fileting' from the outermost erector spinae tissue, separating the whole layer of erectors from the layer underneath it. We could work from lateral to medial. This work would be done if I was focusing on affecting a 'side to side' gait (coronal) issue and bring more sagittal plane movement to the client's gait.

TL Junction: If in your assessment you didn't see movement in the spine in walking, give this area particular focus just as you would the erector spinae tissue.

Quadratus Lumborum: Approach it the same way as above and in the areas between floating rib and ilium. Remember we want ease of movement in the ilium and any work on the QL should reflect that. Work in both sidelying and in prone. One option here would be to bring lengthening to the tissue by having the client tilt their pelvis (posteriorly and anteriorly) as you work the tissue. For example, as you're working in the superior direction, have your client posteriorly tilt their pelvis. This will lengthen the tissue of the lateral side. If you work in the posterior direction, you could have your client anteriorly tilt their pelvis.

It's very important to understand that not only are we working along planes but also within planes

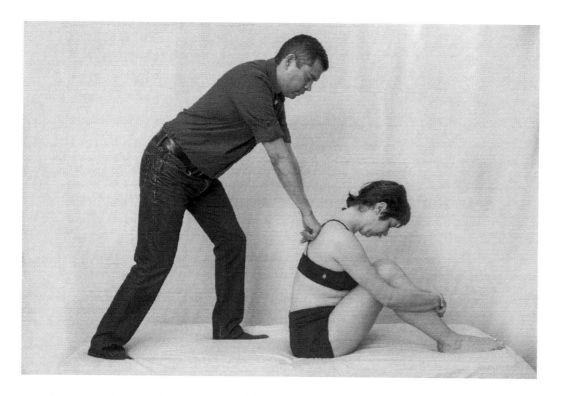

Generally in a session, when working in the pelvic area and then moving up to the shoulders for example, it's important to give the client the sense of connection between the two territories and to let them feel how two different areas relate to each other. 'Striping' down the erectors is one way to integrate the work and to connect the work from two such locations. Use soft fists to go from TL (thoraco-lumbar) junction area down to ilium. This is used in many SI sessions to help the client with integration and is done before asking the client to walk.

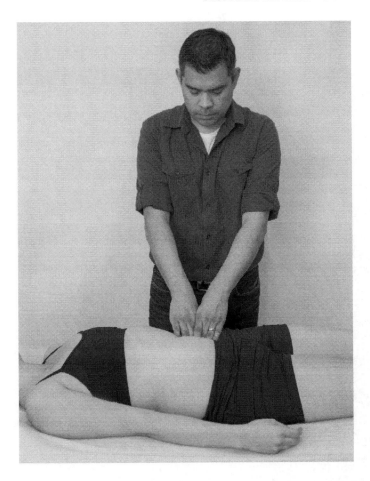

Working the abdominal area now brings to the forefront the work of integrating the client's core. Tight abs or psoas can put strain on the back (think quadratus lumborum) area and prevent movement in the back of the core. A tight abdominal or psoas area can also show up in the anterior neck area and in the upper back area when the client is walking. If you see that (tight anterior neck) happening, then go to superficial abdominals and/or psoas and palpate for tightness.

Abdominals: Holding the rectus abdominus, palpate and 'lift them off', imagining they are being differentiated from the bottom layer. The rectus abdominus muscle can also be moved clockwise or counter-clockwise to determine which direction is tighter. In future chapters we will be discussing goals such as support and capacity that can be affected by working this area. Working the abdominals and psoas allows this part of 'core' the ability to lengthen (in the front) as it is directly affecting the column 'core'. There is also a connection/relationship between abdominals and the front of the cranium. The front of the cranium is referred to as the visceral cranium.

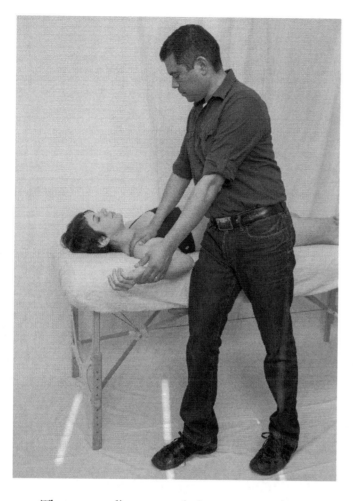

    The pectoralis area and the arms are thought of as areas involved with movement and with breath. Classically, work in this area happens in the early stages of a series and prepares the body for other work. The thinking is that we want to create the ability to move before we provide change or a new movement. Initially, one of the first areas worked on in a series is the breath, the clavicle and first rib. Although Core Integration may deviate from this thinking, I find it a great exercise to feel for space between clavicle and 1st rib and perform clavicle 'play' in all directions early on in a series.

Pectoral fascia: With an open, relaxed palm, move the pectoral area from all directions of that frontal plane and find the area that needs more possible targeted work. Work superficially then deep in this area. Imagine that your work in this area can go from pectoralis tissue to lung and heart fascial bag tissues. You can also work with your ulna as shown in the picture above.

Upper Trapezius: With client in prone, get a grip of the trapezius tissue of the neck with both hands and imagine you are 'peeling' it away from the connective tissue underneath it. Feel for directional resistance, which way does it not like to go? This directional resistance is an indication of possible dysfunction.

    Lower Trapezius: As with the erectors, feel for the edge of the trapezius, 'slicing' underneath the tissue to free it up from adhering to erectors or rhomboid tissue. Imagine how this work could help a client with little movement in their thoracic area during walking.

Triceps: With the client in prone, the practitioner can sit on the edge of the table and bring the client's arm over their own leg and move the tricep tissue around to find the direction of restriction. Note that tightness in the rhomboid area can also be associated to tightness in the rotator cuff/triceps area. Also remember that working in this area is directly affected by work in the latissimus dorsi territory and that particular tissue extends to the quadratus lumborum area. This work can easily be done in side-lying position and when working in that line of tissue, it's necessary to understand how the teres minor and serratus anterior tissue influence how well the arm moves in walking and how well the lateral line of the client is 'expressed' in movement.

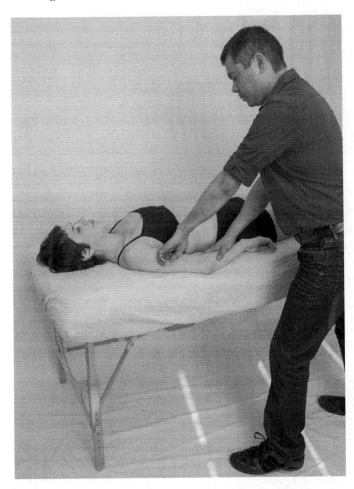

The intermuscular septum of the arm can be thought of as the ilio-tibial band of the arm as it helps to transfer movement down the arm. It can also can as tight and restricted in someone who walks with their arms bent, much like the march of a toy soldier.

Upper arm: Work the fascia that runs down from the deltoid. Just like the ilio-tibial band, the fascia from the deltoid runs down to the lateral epicondyle of the humerus. Working this tissue helps to relieve strain in the shoulder girdle and may help to activate the deltoid muscles if the client is dealing with a 'frozen shoulder' condition.

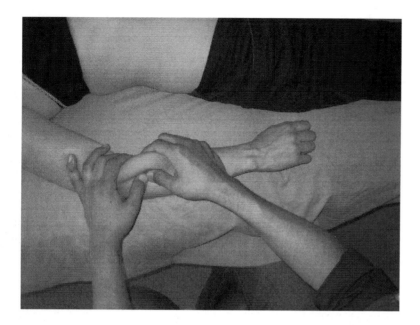

Lower arm: Holding the tissue of the lower arm, move it clockwise and then counter clockwise to differentiate it from the fascial bag below it. Move it in all four directions to find the area of restriction and work that area more. Work in this area gives the client another sense of where they are in space (their proprioception) and aids in bringing more movement to the spine by encouraging more contra-lateral movement via arm swing.

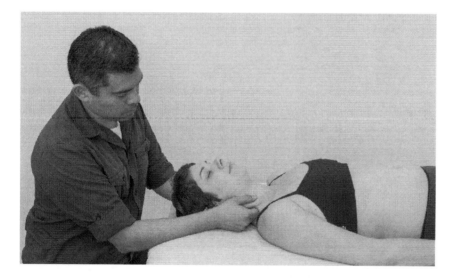

The neck: Accessing the fascia surrounding the sterno-cleidomastoid (SCM) allows you to loosen up the neck without having to work deeply. This move is meant to 'unwind' the SCM as the SCM spirals inward towards the midline. Your work in the neck area is meant to allow for the head to read more clearly information about a more functional way of moving in the rest of the body and should be done after the client is able to integrate this work. This means, the shoulder girdle, pelvic girdle, and feet should be able to be a good foundation for work done in the neck. Is it possible for neck work to be done before shoulder or pelvis work? Yes, it's possible but care should be taken to determine the extent of the work (amplitude).

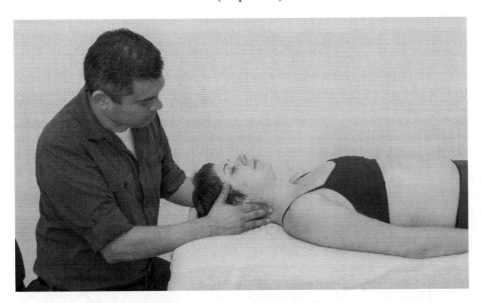

With a couple of fingers, imagine you are 'peeling' away the trapezius from the layer of deeper cervical fascia underneath. You are working in the posterior triangle area.

The head: Holding the head firm, work the fascia of the head by imagining the head covered by a 'helmet' that can be moved around in all directions. Imagine the relationship between this top fascia and the neck fascia and how this can affect folks with a forward head posture.

Closure: It's just as important to know how to leave the client as it is to know how to initially approach the client. Classically, we use a cranial hold or a sacral hold to end a session but with MMCIT we include other techniques that help with closure. These will be covered in future chapters.

Although terms like 'releasing' 'stretching' or 'lengthening' are used when describing what we do to myo-fascial tissue, current findings point to the fact that we don't stretch or lengthen myo-fascial tissue. When seeing these terms when describing myo-fascial techniques, interpret them as 'working' the tissue.

5 MMCIT PHILOSOPHY

Before we dive into the protocol of MMCIT (Morales Method® Core Integration Therapy), I usually do an exercise with my students where I ask them: As bodyworkers, what are our goals with our clients? Inevitably, we come across answers such as: Mobility, flexibility, strength, empowerment, sense of ease, balance, etc. From these answers we discuss and distill a list of strategies/goals that fall in line with those of the Morales Method® Core Integration Therapy. These are as follows:

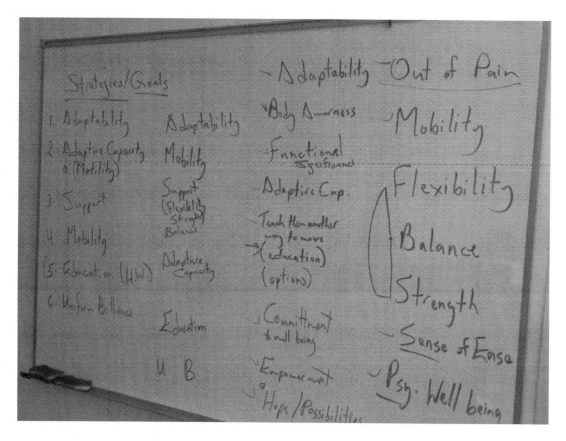

Definition of Goals (in the order of how we address them)

Adaptability- This is described as the client's ability to adapt to changes in their system. Before anything else, this is an inherent place that the client is in at the moment. This may be a factor of the client's body and what has happened to it due to trauma or injury but it could also be a product of their world view, their emotional state, or a habitual pattern. If the client is not able to take on a possible change to their system due to an injury or alteration that is causing them pain, then adaptability addresses their pain and attempts to bring pain relief foremost before moving on to creating a series.

Adaptive Capacity – This is the ability for the client's system/body to take on the work, either in general or in a particular area. In order to create a change or a different option of being/moving, the work on an area needs to be preceded by work that will allow the body to take on said work effectively. With adaptive capacity we as practitioners ask ourselves the question: Can the client effectively respond to the work in this area and if not, then where do we need to go first in order to create the capacity for them to do so? An example of this would be a client with forward head posture who may actually need bodywork in their abdominal area or hamstrings in order for them to be able to fully accept the work done around their neck and head.

Support – This goal seems the easiest for people to understand. In walking/movement, we can clearly see the client responding to gravity and if we need to give them the means to move in gravity (in the vertical position) with more ease, we can easily see how having the musculo-skeletal system 'stack' on itself can provide more support. We can ask ourselves: What order do we need to do our work in order to build on the work we previously did. Almost like building blocks, we seek to 'stack' our work effectively. It's important to not forget that this 'stacking' of our work doesn't necessarily have to always happen from the bottom up. We are multi-plane, multi-dimensional beings and our neuro motor system can create relationships in our musculo-skeletal system that don't always work from the bottom up. It's possible to support the feet by working the pelvis.

Mobility – This is exactly what it sounds like. We seek to bring movement in certain territories and this is usually done by working the myo-fascial tissue. We ask ourselves: How do we bring about functional movement in the body? Where do we need to go (in terms of myo-fascial bodywork) in order to see/feel/experience movement along the proper planes in an orderly fashion?

Education – Inherently, we as bodyworkers are tissue workers but we must not forget that our clients could also react positively to a combination of myo-fascial work and tissue toning/strengthening. Depending on our qualifications, education could be in the form of exercises or movement education. Education could also take the form of helpful information or a referral to another practitioner qualified in another modality/system.

Closure – When working in a series, what's left? With MMCIT we believe that in order to achieve 'happiness' we seek to bring closure to the series and put a nice endcap on the work. This does not mean the interaction between practitioner and client is over but instead there is closure to this series and there could opportunity for another level of work in a future series.

> **"If you analyse the function of an object, its form often becomes obvious"**
> **Prof. F.A. Porsche**

Going back to the words of Jan Sultan, we can now apply the strategies we just described to answer the questions:
1. Where do I go to first?
2. Where do I go to next?
3. How and when do I exit/close this session?

When we combine the strategies and the questions above, we come up with a few guidelines and our order of work becomes concrete. First, we follow these guidelines:
You work the territory that addresses Adaptability and Adaptive Capacity. Then you work the areas that enable Support. Afterwards, you address Mobility. It's only after addressing these areas that you seek to close a session/series by moving towards Education. Finally, techniques are performed to bring about Closure/Integration. Keep in mind that the order of the principles are also meant to meet the goal of Closure/Integration.

Before we can look at how to apply this strategy and philosophy, we need a structured protocol. I will be the first to say that a structured protocol is only as good as your ease and willingness to let it go. When I was going through my martial arts training I was often told that the drilling of basics was done in order to be able to one let it all go and 'play jazz' which entails using intuition and a free flowing mind in order to improvise. It's not reasonable to ask someone to 'play jazz' right away. Instead, the protocol needs to be done over and over again before the practitioner starts to 'get it' and can let it go.

These strategies are very similar to the classic form of Structural Integration but the order of our work is slightly different. Our order differs from other orders of Structural Integration in that with Morales Method® Core Integration particular attention is paid to the core as we see it. The series of sessions in Core Integration also differs from other forms of SI in that we see our work as being compartmentalized in packets of three. This creates the possibility for nine or twelve sessions rather than the classic ten. Nothing is lost in this form of work, we are simply taking a different approach.

Finally, planes of movement are not worked in their entirety in one full session as in some classic SI sessions but rather they are worked as they relate to the territory being worked on and what the body calls for. Planes are worked on in the Order of Complexity and the complexity is based on the client's sophistication in function, how a client may be seen moving functionally (or not) in walking and in other assessment tests. This goes back to our visual assessment.

Previously, we said that we would look at how the body moves along the planes in this order: Sagittal, Coronal/Frontal, Transverse, and Rotation. This order is similar to a baby's stages of motor development and to repeat, we work the planes of movement by order of complexity. **So, this means that we could work with the sagittal plane in mind and eventually with the transverse plane in mind as a practitioner continues to work on a client in a particular territory and increases the complexity of the work. The level of work that deals with rotation would come much after the sagittal level.**

The model for the structured protocol looks something like this except for the fact that inter-osseous membrane work in all limbs can occur in session 1:

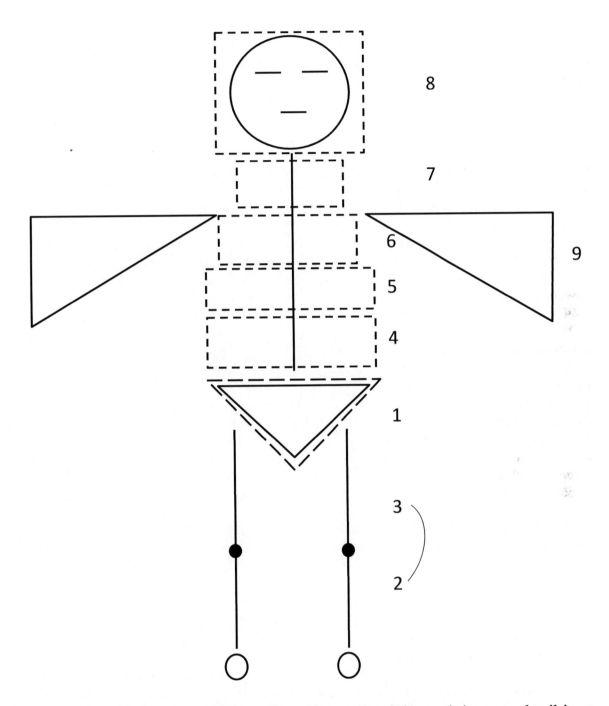

Notice that this model starts with the pelvis. The order of the work in more detail is as follows:

Pre-Session work: This is where we address the principle of Adaptability and help to create the ability for the client to take on series work. This most typically takes on the form of pain relief bodywork. Pre-session work could last anywhere from one to three sessions but of course depends on the client and the severity of the condition.

Session 1: Pelvis. This, according to our philosophy, is where we address capacity, support, and possibly build Adaptive Capacity for future sessions. We work to facilitate movement along the sagittal plane and if there's enough adaptive capacity already in the system in this territory, we move on to other planes. If not, we stay with one plane, and deal with the 'lowest hanging fruit', meaning, the easiest accomplishments to achieve. Superficial as well as deep layers are addressed in this session depending on what the tissue allows and calls for. It's possible that the first session may address the pelvis along the sagittal and coronal plane and future sessions (for example, session 6) may include pelvis work along the transverse plane or with rotation. In addition to pelvis work, this session may include work in the interosseous membranes of all limbs if it's been deemed necessary to do so. One reason to do so is if the practitioner sees a lot of restriction in the area between malleoli and radius and ulna. Working briefly in these areas in session 1 can set up the work for future sessions.

Session 2 and 3: As we recall, we see the feet as an extension of the spine and we work either the legs or the lower legs and feet in order to build support for future work. Support is a main theme of these two sessions. The spine/pelvis is seen as an area that can affect the feet which is why the pelvis is worked first. Afterwards, leg work and feet work follow to provide support for future sessions. Just as before, we work with the Core Integration strategies/goals in mind:

Adaptability
Adaptive Capacity
Support
Mobility
Education
Closure/Integration

If we have enough support in the system we can move to mobility but mobility for mobility's sake can lead to instability. Session 2 and 3 are sometimes interchangeable which is why the figure shows the arrows between leg and lower legs. The practitioner can work on either the leg or lower leg and foot depending on whether or not they have met the Core Integration principles, adding support to future work or creating adaptive capacity for future work. For example, if the bodyworker feels the client needs feet work before moving on to the legs, then the feet and ankles are worked in session 2. The main question an SI practitioner can ask themselves is this: "If I were to work on the leg in session 2, is there enough to support in the lower legs to support the work in the leg?". If not, then session 2 focuses on the lower leg and foot and session 3 moves up to the leg. Answering this question involves visual and palpation assessment.

Session 4: Here we start to work the area that includes the lumbar spine and abdominal core. We continue the work done on the pelvis that contributes to the facilitation of the spinal 'engine'. All planes and all levels of complexity are taken into consideration here but are only worked on if the order of the strategies has been adhered to. This means that if work on the psoas is being done, sagittal or coronal centered work will be done first but work with rotation in mind may be left until later sessions if it's been determined that there is no adaptive capacity to take on that work in this session. How would we know that? This is how I would make that determination: If I saw my client walk and noticed that the thoracic spine was not exhibiting ease in movement I may work the abdominal core in the sagittal, coronal, or transverse planes before addressing rotation. Once I saw that the abdominal work I did is translating into easy movement in the thoracic spine, I may return to the abdominal area in future sessions with rotation in mind. That's what we mean by creating adaptive capacity. Also keep in mind the principle of superficial work and deep work. I may not go to the psoas for example in Session 4 is I run into superficial tissue restrictions in the territory I'm working in. I will want to clear up the superficial restrictions before I work deep in the psoas.

Session 5: This session moves into the area of the thoraco-lumbar junction and can include territory all the way up to T1 vertebra but does not include the scapula and what is classically known as the 'shoulders'. The territory for session 5 further continues with the theme of providing availability for movement (adaptive capacity, support, mobility) in the rest of the spine. If you still need to work with the sagittal plane in mind then work in this area may require you to work with the client in side-lying position and working the outside line territory (for example, the lateral ribs and the quadratus lumborum). You may also need to directly work with the spine by having the client get into extension position (a modification of the yoga 'cobra' pose) or flexed position. This may entail working with the facets and myo-fascial tissue. If you need to work with the coronal plane in mind (based on visual and palpation assessment), then you might be working with the client in prone but with legs off the table to mimic a side bending. As stated before, keep in mind that you could find yourself working with the T-L junction before getting to session 5 but you may not be dealing with session 5 territory on a more complex plane (for example, rotation) until this particular time of the series, session 5. Last but not least, this area addresses superior abdominal work, superficially as it could relate to territory that creates too much flexion in the client (think, costal cartilage), and deeply, as it addresses core abdominal muscles and viscera that affect lumbar spine.

Session 6: This territory can include upper thoracic territory commonly called the shoulders but definitely starts to include scapula work and getting proper function in the arms by working the scapula. Mobility is usually the theme of this session as it would be assumed that enough work has been done in previous sessions to prepare for mobility type of work. Sagittal and coronal plane work is usually pre-dominant in this session and in this case it may include work in the pectoralis and glenoid fossa area. If we have to deal with rotation, then we usually work with ribs and spinal column. In this session we may also start to work with upper ribs that may be inhalation or exhalation fixed.

> ## If we attempt to introduce sophisticated order too early in a series we may end up having to repeat our work later on

Session 7: Cervical work (posterior and anterior) is the main focus of this session. Now that the underlying foundation is set, we want to make sure the 'intermediary' area (neck) between torso and head is transmitting 'functional' information. As with all the sessions, we deal with the planes of movement in their order of complexity. More detail of

Session 8: This session has the potential for becoming more than one session easily as it involves not only head work but also could involve intra-oral work. We usually assume that head work would cover the theme of mobility but when thinking about how many systems 'branch out' from this one area (central nervous system, vestibular system for example) it's possible to see this area as also one that provides support for other areas that deal with movement. When thinking of intra-oral work we should also think of how this area affects the viscera (remember Lion's Breath in Yoga) and how this could tie in to abdominal work from session 5.

Session 9: The arms. Sometimes I think the arms aren't given enough time. They are a peripheral territory in Core Integration but neurologically they are hugely important. For the sake of the structural work, the arms (namely territory beginning from humerus and moving down distally) are left until the end. The arms react to work done in the core and indicate function or dysfunction in the spinal 'engine'. Is it possible to go to arms earlier on? Yes, but we must understand that if we attempt to introduce sophisticated order to the arms early on then that work may fall by the wayside and we may need to repeat the work later on.

A Structural Integration Approach to a Single Session

Before we create a series, it's important to understand how the principles of MMCIT can be applied to a single session. MMCIT and other forms of SI pride themselves on working on a client through a series of sessions and being able to see the cumulative benefits of the work by creating a type of therapeutic relationship that comes from working in a series. Sometimes however it's not possible to see a client for more than a few sessions so it's important to understand how we can help in a single session. Although not ideal, this exercise covers how to work with a client in a single session from a Structural Integration standpoint.

Example: Anterior Shift of the Pelvis

Let's say that we have a client that is coming in for MMCIT series work and is exhibiting an anterior shift in their pelvis. Our first step in describing our work would be to state what we believe some main areas of the body might look like in this scenario. These areas are the same ones we covered in the visual assessment part of this book and we will call these areas, 'hubs'. The 'hubs' could possibly look as follows (keep in mind this is just one possible scenario, don't get too wrapped up in find the one way that people may react to an anterior shift. People are very dynamic and may react differently):

C1/Skull: Anteriorly shifted
T1/Shoulder Girdle: Posteriorly shifted, rounded shoulders
TL Junction: Posteriorly shifted and tight/locked up
Knees: Possibly posteriorly shifted, over extended
Talus: Anteriorly shifted
Medial Arch: Collapsed
Lateral Arch: Tight

We've previously agreed that philosophically, we want to work this way:
1. We go first where we are able to address Adaptability and give Adaptive Capacity
2. We go next where we are able to give Support and Mobility
3. We finish with education and movement work to lead to our goal of closure/integration.

With regards to theory, the ideas we've described build a philosophy for our work but practically, it doesn't tell us where to work. Here is my opinion of how I would work with this scenario along with my thought process. Keep in mind this is a static model. We primarily assess in movement and in movement the body reading/assessment may be different than what my plan is so it's possible that I would come to different conclusions. My opinions here are based on empirical evidence of working with my clients over the years that have exhibited a similar posture/condition.

The Order of Work

1. Initially the first thing that would stand out to me is this person's forward head posture. Secondly, I would notice their anterior pelvis shift.
2. Using Morales Method® Core Integration, I would first look at pelvis and attempt to bring it

more posteriorly. Easier said than done since there's no tight area in the pelvis that when worked can easily allow the pelvis to move posteriorly. Pushing the pelvis posteriorly also doesn't produce much result so what I would need to do is look at the other territories that can affect the pelvis.

3. The other two areas that come to mind are the TL Junction and the hamstrings (they happen to be the areas above and below the pelvis).

4. The TL Junction usually shows up as being an area that is 'quiet' and will most likely show up as an area of LEAST MOVEMENT when walking. The hamstrings will most likely be tight and may restrict any movement I may want to introduce in the pelvis.

5. Under Core Integration the first place I may decide to go to is the TL Junction but I will go there with minimal amplitude (more on this later). I will then plan to go to hamstrings and pelvis and work there with greater amplitude than with the TL Junction.

6. The reasoning behind this is because I want to build Adaptive Capacity for the client to take on the TL Junction work I'd be introducing before I give noticeable Mobility to the TL Junction (Adaptive Capacity precedes Mobility). If I had worked in the TL Junction with great amplitude before I work the hamstrings, I run the risk of giving the client too much movement up top without a base underneath it (remember the pelvis is shifted anteriorly). I therefore need to add movement to the base by affecting its 'tendrils', the legs and feet. Adaptive Capacity and Support before Mobility. Practically this looks like: Hamstrings and Pelvis before major TL Junction work.

7. After working pelvis and hamstrings I would have the client walk and see how they integrate the work.

8. If I see that they integrate the work well, I may go to the TL Junction again and work with slightly more amplitude (remember now your frequency of the work is increasing, since you are working in increments).

9. If I see that they are not integrating the work so well during their walk, then I may go distally and work the distal hubs, like the talus and see if the client needs more support before they can fully integrate the TL Junction work.

10. I may have the client walk and see where they are. If they look like they could still take a little bit more work on the TL Junction I would go there but if they look like they are 'cooked' and say that they feel they are walking 'different' or 'weird' then they are probably done, their system has been altered enough.

11. I may finish off with some minimal work on the shoulder girdle to slightly affect that forward head posture (working the neck and upper trapezius).

12. Again, because of Adaptive Capacity and Mobility, I would only work the posterior neck first, setting up and creating Adaptive Capacity for future neck work (the anterior part of the neck) that would bring about more mobility in the neck.

This is what one session would look like. I may have a plan for future sessions, for example, I may want to further my work on the TL Junction and may want to bring proper movement along the additional planes. If I were to follow the structured protocol I would know what territory to work on with every session but in working a single session I may use the principles as a guide and be open to having the client 'show up', letting their body tell me what to do/where to go with every session.

A quote relating to Adaptive Capacity:
"Preparing the body to receive order precedes establishing order. Changes introduced anywhere in the body must be capable of being sustained and integrated by the whole." Jeff Maitland and Jan Sultan.

6 MMCIT RULES & PERSPECTIVES

Up to this point, we have covered the principles of Morales Method® Core Integration Therapy and have applied them to a scenario to see how we would work. Now we will expand on the previous rules and introduce some perspectives that will help us in understanding the structured protocol.

As mentioned, this work is based on integration of the central core (seen as a cylinder shape) in the body. By integration we say that we are in essence helping to let a core blossom into one that is 'effective, efficient, and happy'. We do this by making sure it has freedom in all its natural planes and operates as close to the 'ideal' as possible within its structural capacity. There are many perspectives of this 'core' in our world, from physical to energetic. We follow and blend ancient knowledge and modern thinking to achieve this. For MMCIT work, two assumptions are made:

1. The arms are peripheral to the core and are worked on last with respect to the order of our work (unless the client is exhibiting a loss of balance/strength or undue restriction in the forearms, in which case the arms and forearms especially are worked on sooner to illicit a more sagittal movement in the arms which thus creates a more tonic engagement of muscles that connect to torso/core (latissimus dorsi, pectoralis major for example). This engages the core incrementally more and creates more of a sense of balance and strength (based on biomechanics).

2. The legs and feet represent an extension of the spine. They can thus affect and be affected by the spine. We work on legs/feet with a vision of how they relate to the spine/pelvis.

If your objective is to integrate the core then we have to start with the foundation of the core, the pelvis. We will make the pelvis our starting point but not forgetting that the feet are an extension of the spine. We strive to make sure all points of the core have functional mobility and stability and have an option to be in their ideal way in all planes.

The planes we want to emphasize and the order in which we want to emphasize them are as follows: Sagittal, Coronal, Transverse, and finally rotational movement. Here's an important thought: Rotation can be seen as the product of the previous three planes.

Amplitude

Ideally, we move up the core. Practically, we may need to work in a different order but we can imagine that our intention is ALWAYS working up the core. Let me repeat: Although our work may take us in different territory, we may ALWAYS be intending on working to affect the core from an inferior to superior direction. This is a key to our way of working.

So would you always work the pelvis first? Yes and no. Practically, no, not if the pelvis is moving sufficiently well. If it is, then follow this rule of movement: Go where you're seeing the LEAST movement or the MOST variation in movement as compared to the plane ideals. This territory is usually the spot that calls out to you the most. We learn to see what is moving the least or varying the most by using the articulation model of body reading and from practicing body reading over and over. To get a different perspective on this, let's imagine the beautiful jellyfish.

When the jellyfish wants to move, it uses jet propulsion. When its body goes through an undulation, the force created by that undulation propels it in the direction its headed. The amplitude of this undulation determines the amount of propulsion. A high amplitude creates a lot of force at the outer rim of the body. Looking at one edge of its body you can see how that undulation may mimic a wave. This wave is inherent at some level in the human body, the core, the spine. Keep this amplitude in mind when we discuss the order of our work. Another way of looking at this idea of amplitude is by looking at kelp in the ocean.

If we observe kelp, the movement of the current moves it in a swaying manner. If we were to move the base of the kelp, you would notice an undulation of the frond/stalk. The greater the movement to and fro at the base (let's call this movement amplitude), the greater the possible movement at the top of the frond/stalk. Imagine that we can create this type of amplitude when we work on a client. If we work too much on an area because we notice that there wasn't enough movement in that area, it's possible to put too much work in the area, too much amplitude. This is what I mean when I say that we can 'amp someone up' or 'deep fry' someone in my courses. What's one way to make sure you don't 'amp' someone up? Make sure we do some work and then get our client to walk around and see how they are integrating the work. When we see them walk we can determine whether they are taking the work well, if they can take more work in that area, or if it's time to move somewhere else. How can we tell that? We look for these signs:

1. The client feeling woozy when getting off the table
2. The client saying that they feel their walk is 'weird'
3. The client has a glazed look on their face
4. Client's pupils dilating or hands/feet get sweaty
5. The client tenses up during the session

The Rule of Increments
When you see an area that isn't moving as well (along a certain plane) we need to ask ourselves, do we want it to be as mobile as possible and as close to the ideal as possible before moving on to a different area? The answer is, 'no'. The reason is the client can seldom integrate our work in one fell swoop, they need time to integrate the work and we don't want to 'amp' them up. None of us welcome a different option of being right away, we need to take 'baby steps' towards a different option of being.

In order to take proper baby steps you need to work in increments. This may involve working the pelvis for example for a little bit of time and then moving up to shoulders (for example) before having to come back down to pelvis. The future work in the same territory can have a higher order of complexity.

What principle is this related to? Adaptive Capacity of course!

Using the Rule of Increments allows the practitioner to build SUPPORT and create ADAPTIVE CAPACITY for future work. Our work needs to be incremental because anything you do will cause 'ripples' and reactions in the rest of the body. You don't want those ripples to be too large so that the client can't integrate them (again, adaptive capacity). If you see an area that is moving too much (varying too much from the ideal line) there's a pretty good chance that there's an area very close by that is not moving at all (or overly tight/taut). That other opposing area is where you would work (the area of least movement). The order of our work and the incremental amount of our work is governed by the previously discussed principles:

Adaptability
Adaptive Capacity
Support
Mobility
Education
Closure/Integration

Breathwork

In many forms of Structural Integration, breathwork is seen as a way to prepare the client for future sessions and to create capacity for future work. Just as it is in the beginning of a yoga session, the yogi preparing their practice starts off with a guided breathwork such as Anuloma Viloma. With MMCIT, we understand that breathwork is an important part of the work and helps the client accept the work and adapt to it. For this reason breathwork is part of every session and not just the first initial sessions. Breathwork's purpose is multi-faceted and its effects are profound:
1. Having the client take a full breath before the practitioner sinks in deeper can allow for the practitioner to access a deeper layer of tissue without causing pain.
2. Having the client take a full breath allows their system to calm down and will allow them to integrate work that may have been a bit intense for them.
3. Having a client take a full breath can be used to bring more body awareness to particular parts of their body. The practitioner can cue the client by saying something like, "go ahead and bring some breath to this area as I work the (whatever territory is being worked).

In the classic method of Structural Integration, just as in traditional Yoga, it was taught that the first session in a series should among other things, emphasize the client's capacity to take in breath as a way to help them prepare for future sessions. In MMCIT, breathing and breathwork is touched on in every session. As a tip, let's not forget that arms and shoulder girdle are very related to breath and breathwork. I believe that breath was a very important starting point for Dr. Rolf because of its importance in Yoga, the Pranayama.

Core Integration Work and the 'Blueprint'

With this type of work it's often said that we 'blueprint' or 'lay down the blueprint' with the aim of working the tissue to 'put things in their place'. If we find through our assessment that a lower leg looks medially rotated for example, and we palpate the area to find that there's directional resistance going in an external rotation, then we would work to restore length in the external direction, assess the client in walking, and in essence, laid down a 'blueprint' of the ideal structure onto the client's 'modified' structure.

Although this method can be extremely effective, it's important to note that this way of working is not without its pitfalls. Firstly, we need to watch that our ego doesn't take over and we work to 'fix' someone by forcing a 'blueprint' on their system. If they don't respond to the 'blueprint' then maybe we're using the wrong approach. Also, we may have all the greatest intentions in the world to lay down a blueprint in order to help our client but if the client's structure is not set up to receive the work (for example, they have bone tissue that broke and healed with a deformation or they were born with a variation in their bone) then the work we may do may actually do more harm than good and our work is fruitless. Keep in mind Monica Caspari's saying, "Happiness is more important than perfection".

Ways of Working Tissue – 'Asking for Movement'

A classic approach by Structural Integration practitioners is an approach that involves getting the client to participate in the work. Dr. Rolf used to call it "Put it in its place and ask for movement". The 'put it in its place' part involves the previous technique of 'laying down a blueprint' in that we take the tissue and the particular body area/territory into the position we believe is a more functional position. The 'ask for movement' piece is exactly how it reads. While we have the client's tissue in a 'blueprint' position, we ask the client to move (flexion, extension, side-bending, rotation, etc.) in order to further lengthen tissue and to lay down a specific sense of where the client's body is in space. Care has to be given when doing this work. We need to ask the client to move in just the right way and along just the right plane or else our work won't be as specific as we need it to be.

We need to minimize confusion and one way is by asking for movement along just one plane (sagittal, transverse, etc.) at a time. Also, we need to make sure we don't 'fry' the client by asking for too much movement. Finally, we need to understand that not all clients are body aware and may not be able to move the way we want them to. Their limited range of motion may frustrate both them and us so we need to do this type of work in increments.

Ways we can ask for movement:

1. Flexion of one or more set of joints along one plane. Flexion and extension of one or more set of joints along one plane when asking for movement will create a more complex movement which will recruit more muscle tissue and will ask for a greater sense of body awareness from the client

2. Rotation (either medial or lateral or both) of one set of joints along one plane. An example of this would be for a client to keep a straight leg while they either medially or laterally rotate it.

3. Asking for movement with the client in sitting, standing, in a yoga pose, or in a pose that is asking the client to exaggerate a more functional position.

Try different ways of asking for movement, 'play jazz' to try to find the best approach for your client. Remember, don't make it too complicated or you run the risk of giving your client information overload.

Ways of Working Tissue – Superficial then Deep Work

Approaching a client and their system will also require you to understand what level you'll be working on, either working superficially or a deeper layer of tissue. When the topic of 'Superficial then Deep' work with regards to working in a series is concerned, it's usually discussed in this way: Before you go deep into a client's system, you want to 'setup' the work by working all the superficial layers/fascial sheets. Only after you work superficially everywhere do you then start to work deeply. This is thought to create a form of Adaptive Capacity (remember that?).

This is a great approach and I believe it not only helps the client to get introduced to the work but also may help with building rapport.

One thing however that has always concerned me about this way of working is that the 'Superficial then Deep' approach may assume the human body is neatly put together in layers. We are in fact much more complex than that. We as systems are not compartmentalized into layers except in our own minds and a tension that may be felt on the superficial layer may be tied to deeper areas either near that area or other territories; ignoring this superficial AND deep relationship during a session (because we were so tied to the dogma of superficial everywhere first, then deep) may make us miss a big part of tension we initially felt. Waiting for future sessions before going deep in a territory, even though you are sticking to a plane, may mean that you need to go back to that territory (and that plane) because you've got unfinished business. To conclude, we approach the 'Superficial, then Deep' method in every session, we don't wait until we work superficially everywhere to then work deeply.

Additional Tissue Technique - The Trailer/Leader Method
Up to now we've discussed using the direct method and using the principle of Directional Resistance to determine what direction to work. Now we're going to add on to that but before we start let's note that the work we've been doing mainly aims to affect the Ruffini mechanoreceptors. These receptors react to slow steady pressure and give the myofascial tissue the cue to achieve 'sol state' and the muscle tissue the possible cue to release. With our previous work we've been working right on the area that we felt needed the work (the 'target' area). Now with this addendum we will be adding a 'leader' or a 'trailer' depending on what we feel works better (i.e. elicits more of a sol state/release). How come this additional way of working? Sometimes creating a 'leader' or 'trailer' is needed in order to get those Ruffini receptors to give the proper release cue. What's a 'leader' or a 'trailer'? The terms 'leader' or 'trailer' will be reserved for work done in front of (the leader) or behind (the trailer) the target area at the same time as target area work (simultaneously)

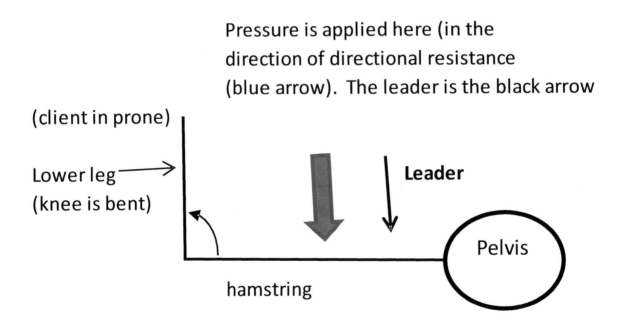

Pressure is applied here (in the direction of directional resistance (blue arrow). The leader is the black arrow

(client in prone)

Lower leg (knee is bent)

Leader

Pelvis

hamstring

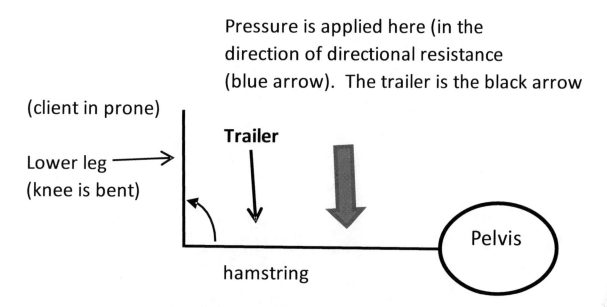

Pressure is applied here (in the direction of directional resistance (blue arrow). The trailer is the black arrow

(client in prone)

Lower leg (knee is bent)

Trailer

Pelvis

hamstring

The concept of a 'trailer' or 'leader' can also be a conceptual one, meaning we may also include limb/appendage or body movement (passive, not active) to mimic a 'leader' or 'trailer'. If this looks familiar to some, we are employing some of the same thinking as used in Positional Release techniques.

The Order of our Work

When we look at a person walk you may be thinking, I want to start at A, then B, then C, then D. Then let's say you go through the session and you only get to A and B. You may make a note for later and tell yourself, "I need to work on C next". When the next session comes around, will you absolutely need to get to C? You may or you may not. The purpose of having your client walk at the beginning of every session includes seeing if there has been any integration or changes to your client in between sessions. Sticking to your pre-prescribed initial plan can be more an exercise of the practitioner's ego than a strategy to help your client. Instead, see your client with 'new eyes' every time you see them walk. They are no longer the same person (It's a fact! We are constantly changing, down to the atom) that they were the last time you saw them.

Don't let this stop you from creating a series or plan in your mind but remember, all things are temporary.

7 MMCIT – FOCUS ON THE FEET & PELVIS

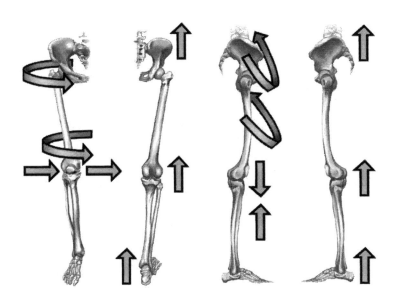

The arrows show possible Directional Resistance in the myo-fascial tissue for the possible scenarios of: Knee shifting medially, High arches, Fallen arches, and Plantar Fasciitis respectively

In order to create a series of sessions when working on a client, we need to be able to see what's in front of us and also be able to imagine what's ahead of us as well as being proficient with the body territories that may present to us in every session. Some of the main areas we need to be proficient are: Feet, pelvis, shoulder girdle, and the neck and head. This chapter will discuss one way of working with lower legs and feet and pelvis.

For a series of sessions to happen successfully we need to imagine (i.e. use our creativity). In chess we think ahead and imagine how one move affects the opponent and how that in turn will affect what we do next. The same applies with this type of work. In putting together a series of sessions we need to imagine how working in one area will affect the client and in turn will affect how/where we work next. Remember the three big questions you will be asking yourself the rest of your life as a bodyworker!

We can use our structured protocol as a starting point for our series of sessions while still understanding that we need to be able to move away from it once we're comfortable with it. Part of our structured protocol involves body reading and the more we do it, we better we get at seeing patterns. Let's discuss the following scenario and imagine the possible patterns. These scenarios are not without variations, differences, and possible contradictions. This is just one possibility of what may happen.

Scenario 1: Fallen Arches

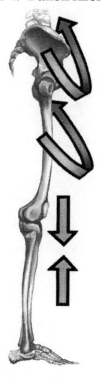

Fallen Arches are a very common, if not the most common scenario you will encounter. Let's imagine the chain of events that can happen (these are just possibilities) by this condition (in movement):

1. Navicular 'meets' the floor at an extreme level, doesn't 'rise' back up. Foot externally rotates in walking
2. Talus shifts medially
3. Tibio-Talar joints bends non-horizontally (possibly more bend at the lateral part)
4. Tibia rotates internally
5. Knee and Femur moves medially
6. Greater trochanter rotates internally
7. Corresponding Ilium inflares

Other than bone, the connective tissue could be short/tight in these areas:
1. Lateral arch tissue

2. Lateral retinaculum
3. Tissue around Tibia/Fibula rotated internally
4. Strain in Pes Anserinus
5. IT Band tightness/taughtness
6. Shortness in Superior Adducters/Pelvic bowl
7. Taughtness in TFL/upper Lateral Rotators, lower lateral rotators could be short
8. Shortness in iliacus area
9. Gluteus maximus could be tight/taut on the superior part of the tissue
10. Deeper glutes (the lateral rotators) could be long and taut on the
superior part and short and tight for the lower lateral rotators
11. Adductors could be long and taut
12. Pubic bone could have a tendency to shift medially
13. The psoas at the lesser trochanter could be rotated medially

Sometimes this type of issue will cause the pelvis to overtly move along the transverse plane. This doesn't necessarily mean there's good movement in the pelvis. It may in fact mean there's LESS movement in the pelvis along the sagittal plane. Let's discuss some general possibilities with other scenarios.

Scenario 2: High Arches

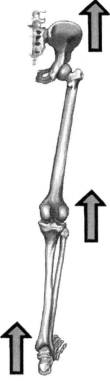

In a normal gait, the arches act as a support (an arch) to take on the weight of the client. When the arches are high and don't release, allowing the arch to come down then back up, there is no opportunity for the normal energy return from tendons and ligaments to occur in the body. This, in my opinion, will not only cause shortness/tightness (in the upper glutes for example) and in other related tissue but it will also cause compensation patterns that will cause improper muscle recruitment and allow some muscles to turn 'off'/not engage (medial quadriceps for example).

Scenario 3: Knee issues – Medial and Lateral

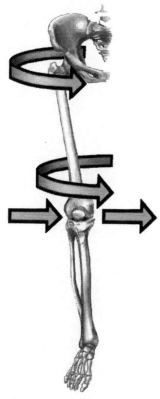

A knee issue can collapse the natural order of the column that is created in normal gait. When the knee shifts medially or rotates medially as a result of this collapse, then other tissue (namely muscle/connective tissue) are called upon to adapt and support the knee, preventing it from buckling. This may result in a walk where we see the knee shifting medially, too far forward, or not being able to extend. The knee isn't built to shift lateral to extremes so if forces push it that way then other bones and muscle tissue 'take up the slack' so to speak and do their best to allow a shift to happen without creating too much strain on the joint. Strain in the muscle tissue can then result. Tissue will either be strained as a result or stay tense as a result or both! Tension is not an isolated incident. Imagine trying to build a birdhouse with cooked spaghetti, that's what it's like to deal with a knee that doesn't support the body.

Scenario 4: Bunions
Bunions can be seen as the body's dynamic way of adapting to a lack of support in the distal part of the foot. This can occur if a laterally rotated foot doesn't fall under the direct line of the tibia or when the distal part of the foot is bound (as in, tight shoes) and the big toe/metatarsal is not allowed to continue the line of force traveling down from the tarsals. These are just a couple of examples. A bunion can affect the foot and rest of the leg in a similar way that fallen arches do. Bunion pain could also result in the client using/over-using other muscles (think, gluteus medius for

example) to swing the leg forward.

Scenario 5: Plantar Fasciitis

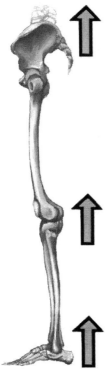

Plantar Fasciitis, a common condition with many of our clients, is something of a 'canary in the coal mine' type of condition. If we pull up a bit and see the big picture, we realize the plantar fascia is the final end of a line of fascia that reaches past the back of legs, up the gluteals, through the thoraco-lumbar fascia, and ends all the way to the skull! Just take a look at Tom Meyer's fascial plane pictures to see this construct. But as we now know, the body doesn't behave in neat orderly planes all the time. Your client's body could be creating a tightness in the plantar fascia not just by pulling up on the plantar fascia from one plane but also from a rotation of the lower leg fascia. When I encounter plantar fasciitis I look not just at the legs but at the gluteals to see if they are allowing for proper movement along the sagittal plane. Most often there is a rotation in one of the legs that is putting an inordinate amount of pull on one or more sides of the plantar fascia.

Scenario 6: Sprained Ankle
For the purposes of this work we can discuss what happens to the client's body when they sprain their ankle rather than what to do for a sprained ankle. A sprained ankle will immobilize the foot, not allowing the normal flexion and extension that happens in gait. When this happens, the client will compensate by swinging their leg out, lifting their leg up, or keeping it rigid with the use of crutches. If the client has been fitted with a medical boot, then they will now have to deal with the stiffness and weight of that apparatus and adapt accordingly. I'm sure there are many other scenarios and ways to compensate. Try to walk around as if you are dealing with a sprained ankle and you will realize what can 'get off the tracks' as far as tissue recruitment and tissue tension is concerned. Once the client has healed from a sprained ankle, there may be some stabilizing tissue

(ligaments) around the ankle that have healed looser than before. This looseness has the tendency to create instability in the ankle and the client will compensate by recruiting muscles not meant for the job or by keeping the foot stiff. This can result in tightness, strain, and a visit to a practitioner such as yourself!

Cycling Pedal Stroke Dysfunction

Let's imagine a cyclist with a pedal stroke where the tibio-talar joint doesn't bend evenly, forcing the knee to go medially at the down pedal. This may cause strain on the medial side of the knee and the client may feel it by the Pes Anserinus area or even by the groin area. This type of pedaling could also cause tightness on the lateral side and could be felt in the IT band or even in the tensor fascia latte or gluteal muscles. I use this example to ask my students: What do you see happening with this client and what would you assume the client may be feeling? How would you tailor a series of sessions for this client? Of course, since this is theoretical we may not all have the correct answer and in fact, there may be no correct answer but it's important to go through this exercise to start envisioning what a series of sessions would look like. Although we may use the protocol in order to create a series, a client with an issue in their knee similar to this may have a series with a certain 'theme' to it, an area with recurring work in certain increments.

The following is a visual collection of techniques that can be used when working the feet, leg, and lower leg. The descriptions for the techniques are mainly meant to depict certain scenarios seen when working with clients rather than explain the full technique. Further explanations occur during the teaching of the program.

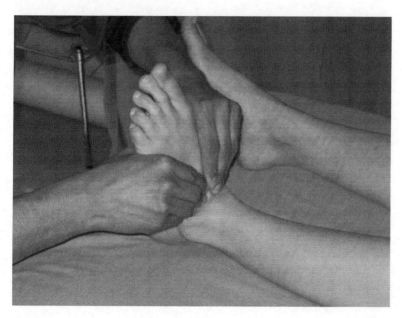

If you notice an uneven/non-horizontal bend in your client's talus, then we can use the same technique we used when we palpated the tibio-talar joint and use it to bring movement to the area of the tibio-talar joint that needs it. Take the joint into dorsiflexion, placing your fingers in the area where there is less flexion.

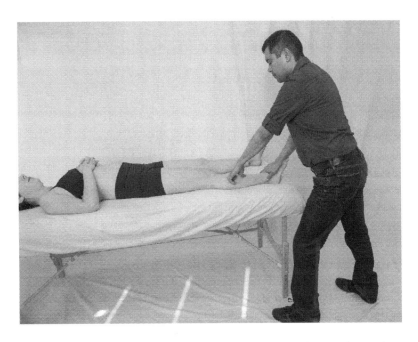

As we see our client walk we may notice more internal rotation versus external rotation in the lower leg. Working the tissue following directional resistance (as in the photo) will help to bring more sagittal movement and more balance in the Screw-home effect of the lower leg.

Working the lower leg either the anterior or posterior territory can be worked in this manner. Again, depending on the directional resistance you could work in either direction (superiorly or inferiorly). Notice I am internally rotating the leg in order to expose more of the anterior leg myo-fascial tissue.

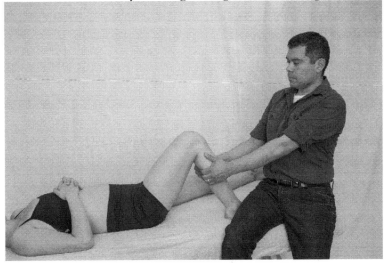

When mobilizing the tibio-talar joint this technique is a deep and effective technique. The key here is specificity. When we previously palpated this area, we could feel for what area of the tibio-talar joint needed work. It may be more in the medial part of the lateral part of the joint. Keeping that information in mind, have the client stand in front of you. Bring your big or second toe in the specific area that needs movement and ask your client to do a slow knee bend. This will add movement exactly where you need it. Your toe may be more medially or laterally depending on the area that needs the work. Hold on to them so they don't lose their balance but don't let them rely on your hold to the point where they are leaning back.

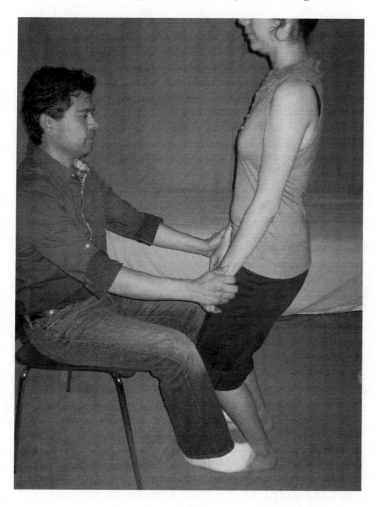

Working the Pelvis

When assessing and working on your client's pelvis, it's important to think about:

1. The different patterns that may reside in the pelvis (tilt, shift, rotation)
2. How these patterns can lead to function/dysfunction in the whole body (dysfunction with regards to movement away from the sagittal plane in walking)
3. Through visual and palpation assessment, a way to discern these patterns
4. How to integrate pelvis work with work in the rest of the body

The pelvis has a unique relationship with the body. The sacrum area has been described as the 'doorway to the fertile underworld of creation' in some studies of anthropology. In the drawing in the beginning of this chapter, you can see a representation of two types of posture. The drawing on the right represents a posture that may be physiologically dysfunctional. We can discern from this drawing how an improper posture may affect all the major areas of the body (the hubs) namely: The arches, talus, knees, pelvis, thoraco-lumbar junction, shoulder girdle/T1, atlas, and skull.

A note on the TL Junction: If you read any literature or Google TL junction you're going to get something like this: The TL junction is the area of the spine by T12/L1. But if you look at the human spinal column, you can see that the vertebrae above the TL junction are not pure thoracic vertebrae. From T8 to T12 you can start to see a change from the pure thoracic to a vertebrae that more resembles T12. SI practitioners call this area the 'functional TL junction'. Keep this in mind when working this area, the structural TL junction and the functional TL junction may be in different areas for your client. A pelvis (in movement) can bilaterally or unilaterally rotate, laterally shift in an unbalanced way, or bilaterally or unilaterally tilt. This can happen in countless angles. A pelvis (in movement) with all its variations can:

Flatten medial arches and/or tighten lateral arches, anteriorly or posteriorly shift the talus, put unilateral (or bilateral) strain on a knee joint, cause a 'stuckness' or a lack of articulation in the TL junction, cause a slumping (protraction) or retraction in the shoulder girdle, cause tightness in the suboccipital area and/or shifting in the atlas and skull, and cause shortness/tightness in the jaw and anterior neck/jaw area (viscero cranium).

As an exercise I have students take turns walking. From there we see what could be happening in the pelvis and how our classmate's pelvis could be affecting the main 'hubs'. Afterwards we verify our findings through palpation of the pelvis and those main hubs.

I tell my students to try looking at their classmates in three different ways:

1. The first way is the way we've been looking at them all the
time, from a head on direction or from one the side of the room.
2. The second way is this: Turn away from them and look at them from your peripheral vision. What stands out to you the most when you do it?
3. The third way is this: Turn your head so that you are facing them head on but with your eyes closed. Open your eyes for only 1-2 second and close them again! What stood out for you as you saw them walking for that brief time, either in their pelvis or another part of their body? Repeat the process and see what happens.

These are different ways of training your SI eyes and visual acuity. Try doing these exercises in everyday life. Sometimes the client's pelvis can have a joint restriction and in addition to soft tissue work we may have to perform joint range of motion techniques.

Time spent in the pelvic territory during a series may include time on enabling the client to move with a more functioning pelvis. This means that work may need to be done with the goal of getting the sacro-iliac joint to move with more fluidity and also possible relieving low back issues. Unlike the chapter on myo-fascial techniques, the following techniques are included here to help with these specific goals (ease of movement and functional ease). When a pelvis is no longer functioning optimally, other areas may over engage to take up 'the slack' or may appear to have 'shut down' (lack of mobility) from over use. Imagine a client walking with a pelvis that lacked some movement along the sagittal plane and instead it moved more along the transverse plane. Now imagine that their thoracic spine is completely still and they may be also complaining of discomfort in their thoracic spine. It could be possible that the thoracic spine (and quite possibly the shoulder girdle) at one point in time worked overtime to get the client moving and discomfort in their thoracic spine is due to an overworked territory. The following techniques are meant to help with assessing a pelvis and working to get the pelvis more functional.

The SI joint is shaped like a kidney bean in the area is that can be most affected by our work and moves along on this curved 'track' on both sides. Because of this, normal movement of the sacrum in walking exhibits a rotation along the vertical axis and movement superior to inferior along the SI joint. Imagine the sacrum moving like a royal 'wave' when a client is walking. Try this as an exercise: Have your client walk in front of your while you have your thumbs on their sacral base. Have your hands on their ilium as you're doing so. See if you can feel the sacrum move while the walk. Maybe you can feel your right thumb (on their right sacral base) move anteriorly as they take a step forward with their right leg. If so, this the natural movement of their sacrum. If you're not feeling this movement and if you see your client move with that one side moving as a 'whole', without articulation along the sagittal plane, then it's possible that the SI joint could be restricted.

Understanding the lumbar vertebrae

The main thing to remember when working vertebrae is that there is movement (rotation) with the vertebrae during spinal movement (side-bending). This is a basis of Fryette's Law.

When the spinal column side-bends to the right, the thoracic and lumbar vertebrae will rotate counter-clockwise (as seen superiorly from the vertical axis above and assuming neutral position). When the spinal column side-bends to the left, the thoracic and lumbar vertebrae will rotate clockwise. Knowing this will help you with misaligned vertebrae and getting a 'stuck' vertebrae to move.

FIRST LAW: When the spine is in neutral, side bending to one side will be accompanied by horizontal rotation to the opposite side.

SECOND LAW: When the spine is flexed or extended (non-neutral), side-bending to one side will be accompanied by rotation to the same side.

THIRD LAW: When motion is introduced in one plane it will modify (reduce) motion in the other two planes.

Assessment

In general, we want to assess and palpate all of these areas for evenness and movement. Once we find something that may be out of alignment, we work that area to bring balance and then re-assess for balance and pain.

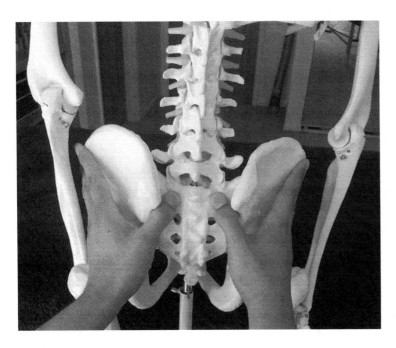

All Areas we can assess:

* Sacrum/ SI Joint
* ASIS
* L5 and other Lumbar Vertebrae
* Pubic bone

Assessing Sacrum
1. Check for nutation in sitting or in standing during flexion
2. Check for movement in walking
3. Check for torsion in prone and for upslip/downslip in prone

Possible Findings
1. The more restricted side doesn't move as much in walking
2. The restricted side moves superiorly in standing flexion test
3. The restricted side doesn't nutate properly in sitting test
4. The restricted side won't move as much in prone test (inferior move)
5. One ILA (Inferior Lateral Angle) is more inferior than the other

Assessing Lumbar vertebrae
1. Check for rotated vertebrae via the spinous processes while client is seated and in flexion (client curls forward)
2. Check for rotated vertebrae in prone (running fingers along spine)
3. Check for rotated vertebrae in standing (visual assessment while client stands and curls forward)

Possible Findings
1. A spinous process that is more prominent on the left (for example, when palpated with client in

prone and fingers are on each side of the process) could indicate a clockwise rotation of the vertebrae and a vertebrae that is behaving as if it's side-bending to the left

2. A spinous process that moves to the left or right when client is standing and flexes forward could indicate a rotated vertebrae

3. If tissue moves more superiorly on one side than on the other side when client flexes forward this could indicate tissue restriction possibly coming from joint/bone restriction

Assessing ASIS:
• Palpate both ASIS to see if one is more superior than the other or more anterior than the other. This is usually done in supine position (on table) but we will be doing this in standing position first to get a vertical baseline. Only assessing in supine gives you one dimension of the situation.

Possible Findings:
• An off balance in the two ASIS's could be a result of sacral torsion/pelvic torsion. This torsion can be a result of short and tight muscles (such as the quadriceps) or long and tight muscles such as the hamstrings. An off balance can also be the result of weakness in the glute complex (gluteus medius, minimus). Finally, an off balance can be the result of a compensation due to a rotated vertebrae.

Assessing Pubic bone:
• We assess pubic bone with the heel of our palm. We approach the pubic bone by moving superior to inferior on our client. Always check in with the client before you go here and while you are there as this is a sensitive, guarded area for people. If the client is not open to getting work here, not a problem, don't do it.

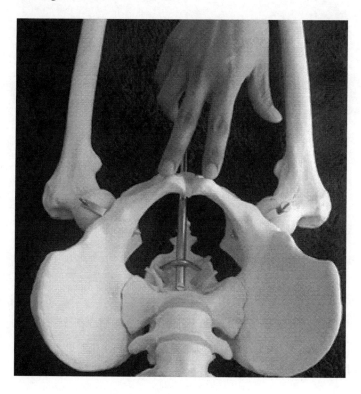

We check to see if one side of the pubic bone is either more posterior/anterior or superior/inferior or medial/lateral than the other

Possible Findings
• A strained side of the pubic bone may feel more sensitive to the client. Further palpation of the adductors attaching to the sensitive side may reveal strained muscle tissue
• A more inferior pubic bone may be accompanied by sacral torsion/SI joint restriction either on the same side or on the other side

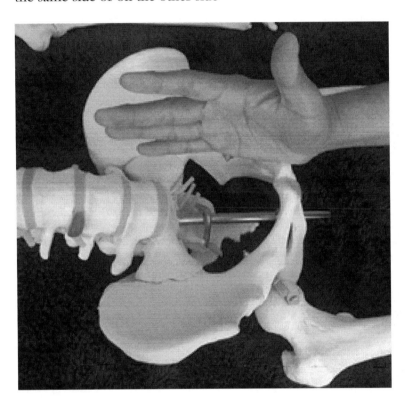

Remember - Assessment can already be seen as therapeutic

Also remember, as you keep assessing clients over years, you will pick up on patterns. Don't be tied to creating causal relationships in your mind.

Working Protocol for Low Back
We will be using the following protocol when working the low back. This is not the gospel as far as working the low back, this is just the way I work and the way I've gotten positive results the majority of the time. Keep in mind that this way of working is submits to the protocol, meaning, we would not work with rotation if we have not resolved restrictions in the sagittal plane.
1. Assess
2. Work the soft tissue
3. Work the connective tissue (in this case, joint range of motion)

4. Perform MET (Muscle Energy Technique) tissue work
5. Perform nerve work (next order of bodywork)
6. Give body conditioning 'Homework' to strengthen weak tissue

Working the Sacrum/SI Joint - Soft Tissue Techniques:

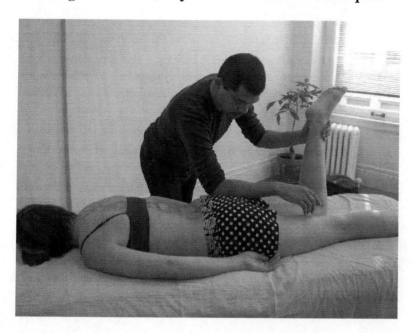

The piriformis can be worked in many different ways. Here I am leaning into it with my forearm as I move the model's bent leg towards me. This lengthens the piriformis while it's also being lengthened by my leaning. The piriformis affects the sacrum since it is attached to the anterior part of the sacrum. Unilateral tightness/shortness can lead to sacral torsion. Overall tightness of the piriformis muscles can also cause flexion of the sacrum.

The Sacro-Tuberus ligament runs along the same line as the hamstrings. If hamstrings are tight, this tightness can run up the sacro-tuberus ligament and cause tightness in the sacrum, causing lack of mobility. If sacro-tuberus ligament is worked to affect the sacrum, then hamstrings should also be worked. Sacro-tuberus ligament work can entail a slow and steady sinking in of the tissue. Similar work as was done on the piriformis can also be done here. Use your forearm to sink past gluteal muscles and approach the sacro-tuberus ligament.

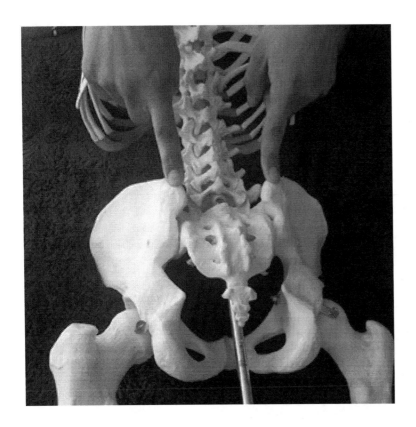

Joint Range of Motion

Working the sacral base of the sacrum in prone, we cup the PSIS with our palms and move inferiorly. The more restricted SI joint won't move as easily. A slow steady pressure is key here.

• Move off from one side to the other of your client in order to eleminate the possibility of a false positive reading and to ensure your pressue is going directly inferiorly

• This is NOT a downward pressure (meaning, going from posterior to anterior). The direction of work is in the inferior direction. Doing a downward pressure could cause injury to your client!

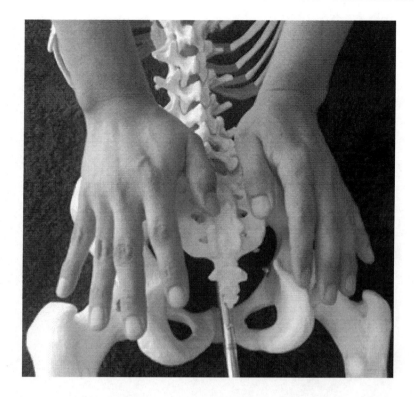

Joint Range of Motion (continued)

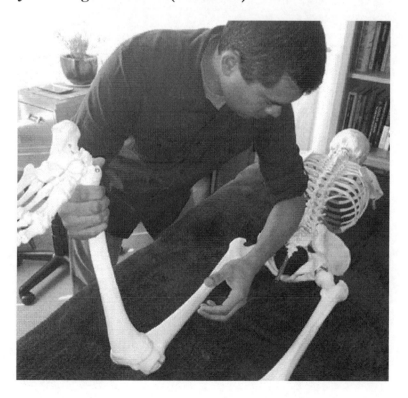

• Gapping the SI Joint, although may look like working the piriformis, is actually meant to create a slow steady wedge between sacrum and ilium. Here I am facing away from the client in order to properly place a forearm in the wedge position

• Direct SI Joint range of motion in supine (bottom photo) entails bringing one hand under the client with fingers right at sacral base. It's important to have the fingers as high up as possible in order to get proper movement of the kidney bean SI joint. Place your other hand over the ASIS and slowly bring the ASIS in a curved trajectory while keeping the sacrum still. This will encourage the articulation of the SI joint along the kidney bean shaped 'track'. Slow and steady wins the race here

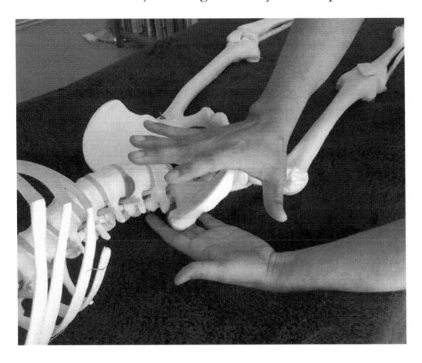

• An alternative to this movement is to work from the opposite side of the table if you are feeling your body mechanics require it

• It's important to imagine the joint and to imagine you are bringing range of motion to the actual SI joint

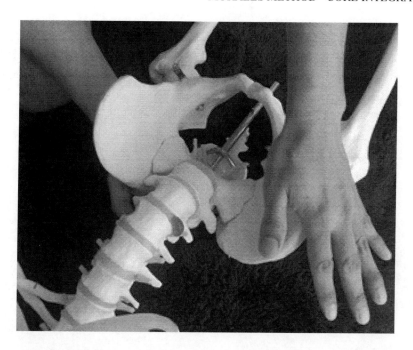

"What is its biological birthright?"
Bruce Schonfeld

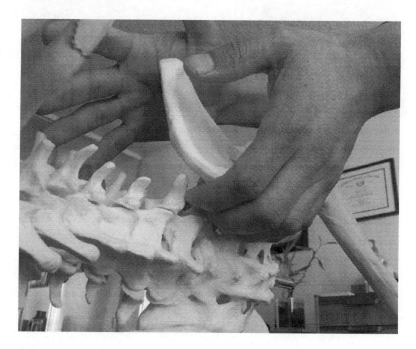

Joint Range of Motion in Standing

• The main objective is still to get the SI moving and here we use gravity and the client's own body to get it to move
• With a thumb on the restricted sacrum side, wrap your forearm around to support your client.

I place my hand and forearm on their ASIS
•   Have your client bring up the knee on the same side as the restricted SI joint. As they do so, support them so they don't fall. Also, create a barrier to motion by going ANTERIORLY so the sacral base doesn't go posteriorly. This will force the SI joint to articulate.
•   Have them do the motion slowly and hold it. Then, have them lower their leg back down. When doing so, create another barrier to motion but this time going Posteriorly/Inferiorly.
•   If the client experiences pain, ease up on the pressure. This is meant to create movement in the SI joint, not to cause pain
•   Thumb placement is important here or else you will not be causing any SI joint movement. Make sure you are at the sacral base

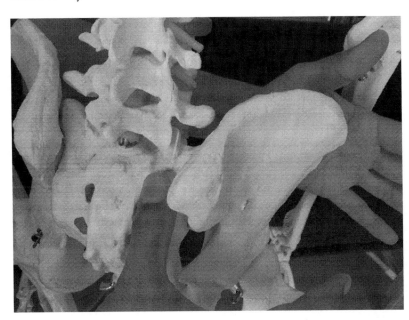

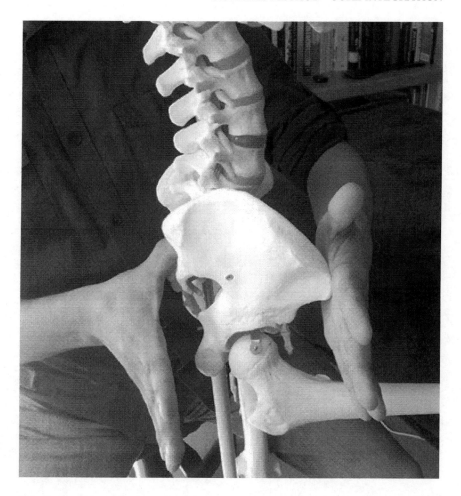

Working the Lumbar Spine

Soft Tissue Techniques - Specificity is key in working the pelvis. Detailed work on the glutes can include Gluteus Maximus, medius and minimus. When working the deeper glute muscles, intend to sink deeply to approach the glute medius and minimus.

Working the quadratus lumborum is effectively done in sidelying position. The small area of space between the floating ribs and the ilium has enough room for two knuckles or fingers. You are essentially working the tissue anterior to the erectors, which is the quadratus lumborum muscle.

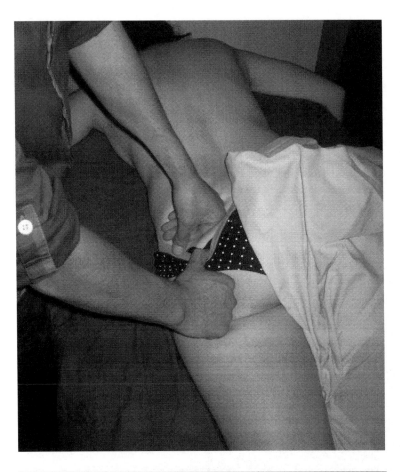

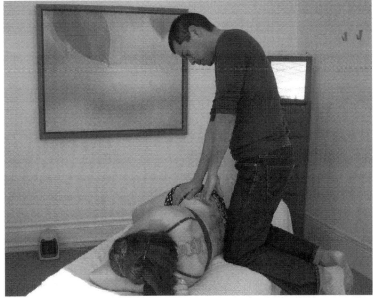

84

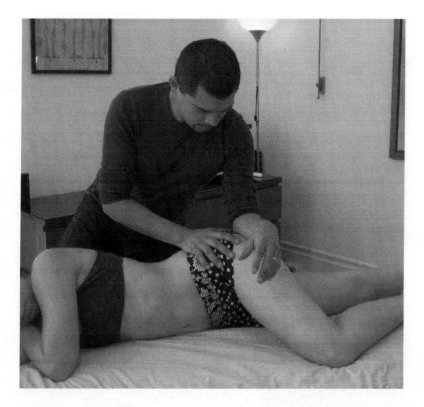

When working with a rotated vertebra, it's important to understand that the rotated bone has a distinct relationship with multifidus and rotatores muscles. Understanding the direction of these muscles will help you determine the direction of your work. For example, if a vertebra is rotated clockwise, then the multifidus on the left hand side could be short and tight and in need of lengthening. The multifidus on the right hand side could be long and taut.

Normally, psoas works is done in this way: As you slowly sink into the tissue, you can ask your client to slowly raise and lower their knee in order for you to make certain you are on the psoas. You can also ask your client to internally rotate their leg in order for them to feel where you are and for you to access a different part of the psoas.

Another way to work on the psoas is to sink into the psoas tissue and move the client's leg out as you are in the psoas. This can stretch the psoas near the attachment of the lesser trochanter. Psoas work can also be done in side-lying position.

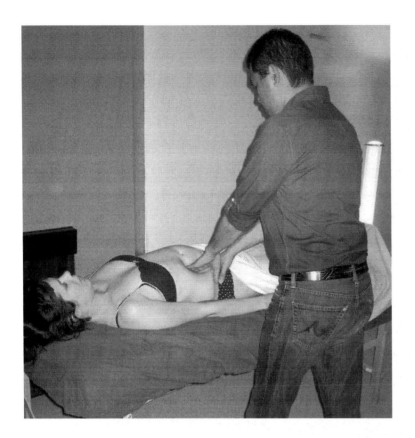

In order to bring relief to the pelvis/low back, work the lateral rotators and all tissue around the greater trochanter to allow for movement in the pelvis, more specifically, movement along the sagittal plane.

Lumbar Joint Range of Motion:

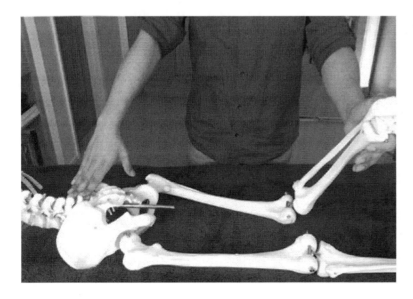

- Besides soft tissue techniques that enable the lengthening of multifidus and rotatores, we can aim to de-rotate a rotated vertebra by using the anchor and lengthen method
- Find the rotated vertebra
- Place your fingers on the shortened tissue next to the rotated vertebra. If a vertebrae is rotated CCW for example, you would place your fingers on the client's right side.
- Bring client's foot up, knee in flexion (approximately 90°)

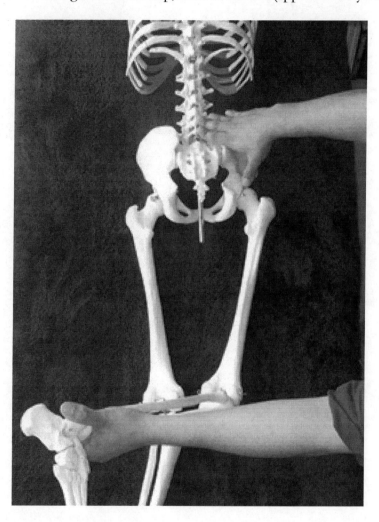

- Bring the foot towards the midline. This will outflare the pelvis and rotate the sacrum, thus de-rotating the vertebra (in the case of the example, more CW)
- Keep your fingers in place, creating a barrier for movement
- When you slowly bring the foot back out laterally, keeping the barrier will help to let vertebra stay in its neutral position and also lengthen short/tight tissue
- Repeat 3-5 times
- Can you see the potential for other moves and modifications with this move? For example, you can put the client in frog leg as you work with knuckles or forearm
- Remember, NOT to move in a downward (anterior) direction. Doing so could injure your client. You really want to work in an oblique angle, to lengthen the multifidus muscles

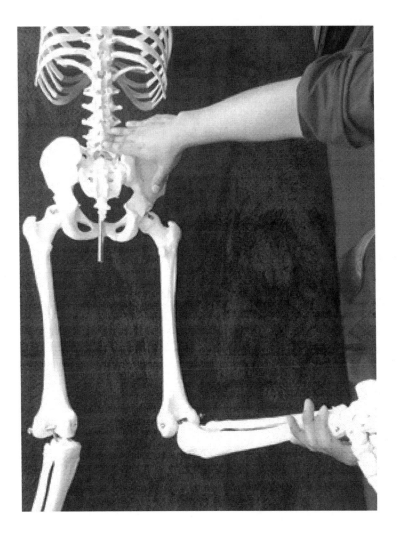

"We specialize in not specializing"
Bruce Schonfeld

Joint Range of Motion (continued):

•   In the bottom photo the client may have a clockwise rotated vertebrae and is lying on his right side, left side up
•   As the vertebrae is clockwise rotated, I would be able to palpate the spinous process of the rotated vertebra much easier in this position
•   My fingers attempt to lengthen the multifidus and rotatores muscles as the client is slowly twisting of their own accord
•   My left hand is on the client's leg only to stabilize myself
•   Note: We are NOT twisting the client ourselves. The client must move on their own and find what feels comfortable for them
•   Can you see the potential for other moves and modifications from this move? Maybe asking for extension and flexion? Understand Fryette's laws to see the possibilities.

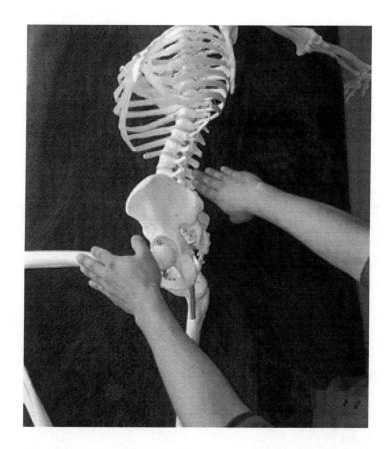

Joint Range of Motion – Psoas

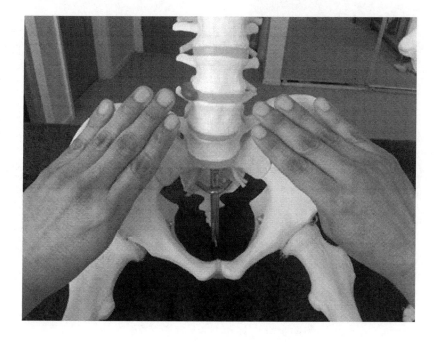

• A lot of techniques for rotated vertebrae of the lumbar spine focus on the posterior part of the spine but this technique affects the back from the front
• With the client in sitting position (knees at the edge of the table)
• NOTE: The picture shows my hands with palms down but for the actual technique I will be having my palms facing each other
• When you feel you are in front of the rotated vertebrae, then have your client lean forward (straight back) as you create a barrier with your fingers
• `You may be feeling the rotated vertebra bump up against you. Move to lengthen the psoas that's most likely tight, right at your fingers. After doing this move then re-assess to see the effect

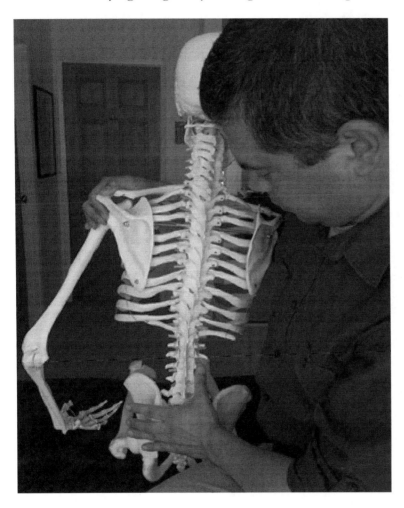

• In this next move, we are taking the vertebra through ranges of motion by having the client flex, sidebend, then rotate.
Find the rotated vertebra and place a thumb near spinous process. Let's say in this example Mr. Otto's vertebra is rotated counter clockwise
• I would hold the client's shoulder to prevent them from falling forward
• I would then help them flex, sidebend to the left, then rotate clockwise. All the while my thumb is aiding in the lengthening of tissue that may contribute to the rotation of the vertebra

- Slow and steady wins the race here
- Can you see the potential for 'playing jazz' here? Maybe working in standing, maybe working with the transverse process instead of the spinous process? However you work, make sure you are checking in with your client throughout the process

Working the Pubic Bone

Soft Tissue Techniques - The Pubic Bone can be pulled into a shear by addcutors and can be pulled out of midline by obturator muscles.

The obturator internus acts as a 'hammock' for the pelvis. Notice how the pelvis seems to hang from this muscle as it attaches to the femur. Also notice the ramus underneath the obturator. The ramus is the point of attachment for adductor muscles and the gracilis. Tightness in these adductors can also affect the way the pelvis moves and can make the pelvis be 'clamped' down by tight adductors.

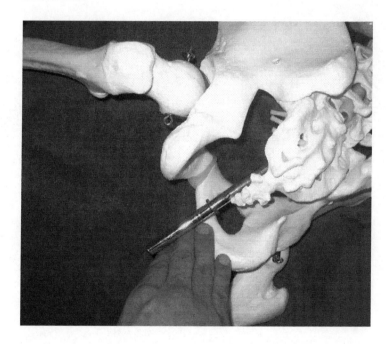

The ramus of the pubis is the area where adductors and the obturator internus attach. Before working this area, ask your client to lift up the leg by the corresponding obturator so they can feel the adductors firing. This will let them know exactly where you're working.

Once the ramus is worked, working the obturator internus requires moving deeper into the ramus and working the other area of the bone. Slow and easy sinking into the tissue is required. This work can help with the client's sensation of tightness in the pelvis area.

Shortened hamstrings can bring about posterior tilt on the pelvis and can aggravate the low back. Working the hamstrings in order to lengthen them can help the low back. Here, I am performing a 'facilitated lengthening' stroke on the hamstring. Since I am close to the ischial tuberosity, I am lengthening a longer part of the hamstring. Note that once I anchor on the tissue, I then lower the leg in order lengthen the tissue. I could opt to work in the opposite direction based on Directional Resistance.

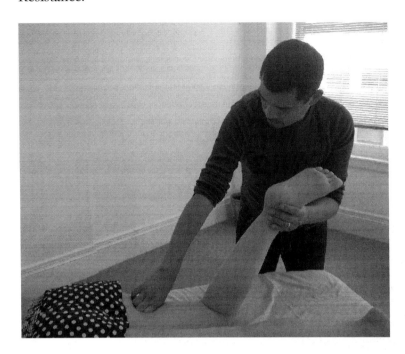

Joint Range of Motion

•   Similar to the work on the SI joint, work the pubic bone by feeling which side may be more superior, inferior, anterior, posterior, medial, or lateral than the other. How do you know which is more posterior or which is more anterior? We may have to feel for d.r. to help us determine that

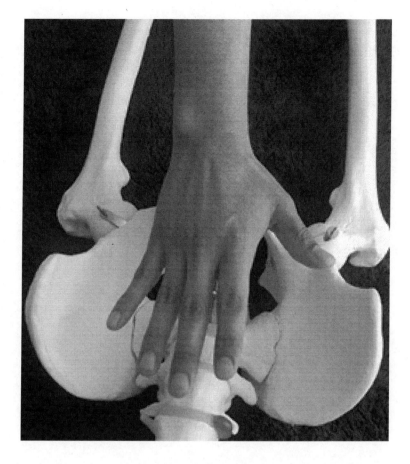

• There is a protocol to this work. The pubic bone is usually the last place we would work at. First address the sacrum to free up any SI joint restriction, then assess ASIS (in standing) to determine soft tissue tightness that may be creating a pull. Then assess pubic bone in supine

• Assess in walking by first checking anterior to posterior shearing (doing a visual assessment). Then check for pubic lateral shifting (again, by doing a visual assessment)

• Then have client in supine position. Place heel of the palm on the pubic bone and slowly, methodically, mobilize the joint in the direction you want it to go, feeling for directional resistance

• Return to the soft tissue techniques if necessary

During the Core Integration 2 program we run through an exercise. We break up into teams of three or four and we imagine answers to how the pelvis could be moving under these possible five scenarios:

Anterior Shift, Posterior Shift, Anterior Tilt, Posterior Tilt, Unilateral Torsion (rotation)/Unilateral tilt (Anterior or Posterior).

From these five scenarios we create possible expanded scenarios (in walking) for the following hubs: C1, T1/Shoulder girdle, TL junction, knees, talus, medial arch, lateral arch. We ask ourselves: What could be going on in these areas during movement?

To prime the pump so to speak we go through the example of the anterior pelvic tilt. We can imagine that following is possible:

1. C1 – Anterior Shift

2. T1/Shoulder Girdle – over flexion, dowager's hump?
3. TL Junction – Possible tighness, anterior shift
4. Knees – Over flexion
5. Talus – Anterior Shift
6. Medial Arch – Collapsing
7. Lateral Arch - Tight

Your Turn!

Try to catch someone walking around (airports are great for this) that is exhibiting an anterior pelvic tilt. See what you come up with regards to those areas. Then, imagine what a session would be like as far as assessing their pelvis and what the possible findings would be. From there imagine what a session would look like as far as how you would work the tissue. If you are feeling adventurous, then imagine what a series of sessions would look like and how you may follow the protocol but create a theme for your client based on what they bring to the table.

8 MMCIT – FOCUS ON THE NECK & HEAD

The neck is a fascinating part of the human body. In our culture and in our expressions the neck has made itself clear as an exclamation point to our meanings. We say things like, "Grab it by the throat" or "Go for the jugular" or "They're neck and neck!" to communicate the importance of some event or action and we use the neck as a method for that expression.

The examples are numerous and they all point to one thing: When we want to underscore something we use body parts as part of our expression. Even the actions that happen inside the neck area are used. Think about phrases such as "I got a lump in my throat" or "swallow your pride" to be convinced.

If you bring your middle fingers and two thumbs around your neck you can see that you can very easily put your hands around your neck. In that small space, that space enveloped by your hands, a myriad of activity happens. We have bone, blood, our central nervous system, lymph, food, water, and air in the form of our breath and our voice all passing through that one major area. It's no wonder so many of us are fascinated by the neck!

> There is a lineage to this work, and it has been influenced by "….a small mystery school whose discipline was a specific form of inquiring into human form and function" Peter Melchior, The Guild for Structural Integration

The following techniques have been collected to be able to clear up issues in the neck when working with your clients in a series. What I usually show in a workshop is how to work with soft tissue in a way that will allow connective tissue (in this case, bone) find its way back into proper alignment. In many cases, improper cervical spine alignment will need to be addressed as we progress in the Morales Method® Core Integration series. The following techniques are meant to be done methodically and slowly, never fast or with any type of thrust. If in doubt, consult a Morales Method® Certified Instructor.

The order of strokes shown here are meant to take the client from general to more precise work. Use your judgment when deciding when to use a technique from the overall repertoire. The techniques are put together using the following thought process:

1.   Preparatory work – The beginning strokes are meant to introduce yourself to the client's neck,

assess any vertebral rotational issues, and formulate a game-plan/strategy

2.   Deeper work – The subsequent strokes are meant to start working on the different areas of the client's neck to be able to address deeper areas of tension and also to be able to work the anterior part of the neck as that may affect the posterior neck

3.   Spinal mechanics work – The techniques in this section are meant to work the soft tissue and to perform slow methodical movements on the cervical spine that allows the cervical spine to find proper alignment. The soft tissue techniques in this section allow for the de-rotation of rotated vertebrae by taking cervical spine joints through specific range of motion movements.

4.   Closing work – These closing techniques are meant to 'say goodbye' to the neck area and bring a close to the session in a relaxing way.

Keep in mind however that when working in a series you may want to pull out the techniques that work best for that particular client at that point in time. If you are working later in the series and working the neck and head area, then the order or complexity will dictate to work to free up movement in the sagittal plane first. As you move through the Order of Complexity you will likely create your own repertoire of strokes, finding the way that works best with you and your clients. Above all, it is paramount that you keep communication open with your client. If a stroke or technique does not feel right to your client, then don't do it. There's always another way.

You are learning to work the neck and head as part of a protocol and we could help a client's neck by working their neck but we could also help by working their legs or their talus (as an example).

We've have accepted this way of thinking, which is great, but also keep in mind that the relationship can move in the other direction. For an example of this, just notice what happens to your hamstrings (back of legs) when you jut out your head, extending your neck out.

I'm often asked in a workshop, "should I work up from T1 to C1 or the other way around?" I have often worked from the ground up so to speak but I urge you not to see the whole world as a protocol. Listen to what the client (verbally and non-verbally) has to tell you and act accordingly. I have also gotten the 'gut feeling' to go straight to their C1 (Atlas) and have noticed remarkable results.

Directional Resistance – Don't forget that directional resistance will determine how you work. Also keep in mind that the planes of movement will dictate which directional resistance you will 'listen' to first and which one you will go to next. We are not devoid of variety. If you need to work in a different direction due to palpating a different directional resistance, then please do so. What is Directional Resistance? This is the palpatory sensation you receive when you take connective tissue in different directions and you feel the tissue does not move as easily in one or more directions. If there is more resistance going in a certain direction, that's Directional Resistance (dr). Working tight tissue (in some cases short and tight, in others long and tight/taut) by taking it in the direction that it is resistant/tight is called the Direct Method.

As with Deep Tissue Bodywork, these techniques are meant to be slow and methodical, allowing your hands to sink into the tissue as the exercise most of us have seen/done with a bowl of corn starch and water.

TECHNIQUES - Preparation Work

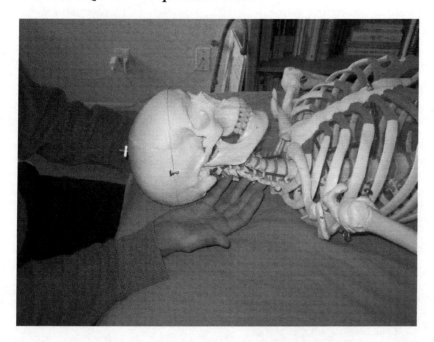

Striping of the neck - This movement is meant to assess the muscles of the neck and to help formulate a plan for further work. We move from the T1 area all the way to the occiput. Notice the table is used as a fulcrum to allow for minimal wrist usage. The striping does not involve lifting up

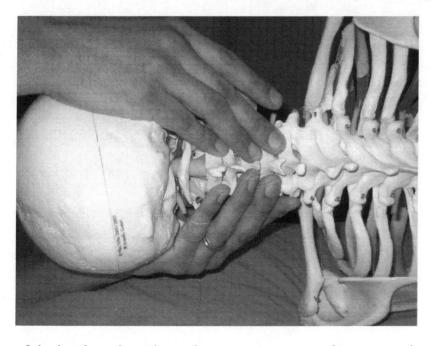

of the hands at the wrists rather you can use your forearm as a lever to allow your fingers to work the soft tissue between the Transverse Process (TP) and the Spinous Process (SP), the lamina groove. The next photo (above) shows a different view of the same striping technique but don't confuse it with a technique. We are NOT putting the client in side-lying position for this technique. With my fingers in this position I can feel for trigger points, a vertebrae that is rotated, and tight superficial (upper trapezius, splenius) myo-fascial tissue. I can also palpate for tight connective tissue septums.

The movement can vary as follows: Both hands moving inferior to superior at the same time or alternating (one hand moves up then the other, as the first hand moves back down to the T1 area to repeat the process). Note that in the first photo I am keeping the skeleton's head in neutral position. The movements are minute and I only move as far as a vertebrae or two for the sake of precision and assessment. Keep in mind how this technique can help assess and treat tissue that is dysfunctional in the sagittal plane.

When working the trapezius and occiput, be sure to move out laterally away from the cervical spine. This ensures a cross fiber stroke on the trapezius tissue that attaches to the skull. The head is

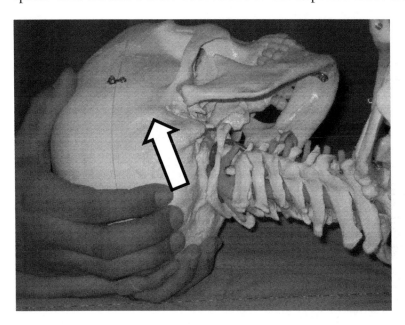

NOT turned to the side for this technique. I'm doing it here for illustration purposes only. I will usually alternate the strokes (one side then the other) in order to be able to support the client's head better. In addition to moving medial to lateral, this stroke can be modified to primarily work on the Sterno-Cleido Mastoid attachment at the skull and can be worked in a lateral to medial direction. Keep in the mind the direction of your technique will depend on Directional Resistance. Slow and steady work in this area is great for releasing tight tissue and/or trigger points.

Thumb work on the lateral side of the neck going towards the feet (inferiorly), is a great way to work the multifidus and the other cervical spine muscles that run along the lamina groove.

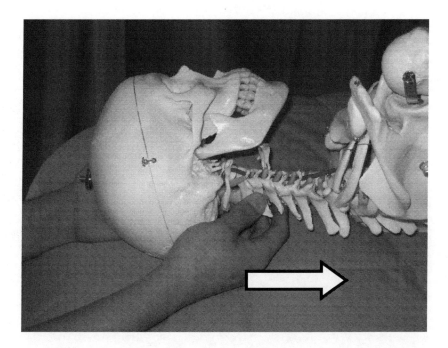

This technique can be lightened up to use it as a 'preparatory work' move or the force can be increased for deeper work, if necessary. Because I'm using their bone to 'sandwich the tissue', a strong barrier is created and very little force is necessary to create deep work, thus less strain on your thumb joint. To create more force, move your hand so that you create almost a perpendicular angle between thumb and neck. Check in with your client to make sure the pressure is not too great as there is potential to create a lot of force in this manner.

You can also work going in the superior direction if the directional resistance calls for it. These two techniques can also form the basis of spinal mechanic work later.

Even though you may feel directional resistance going inferiorly, make sure you finish working inferior to superior. This ensures you finish the work with encouraging space between the vertebral facets. Don't forget about the sub-occipital muscles and working them in this direction with the thumb tool. This technique could be very effective on the Rectus Capitis Posterior Minor tissue. The next order of work with this technique would involve client participation (head movement).

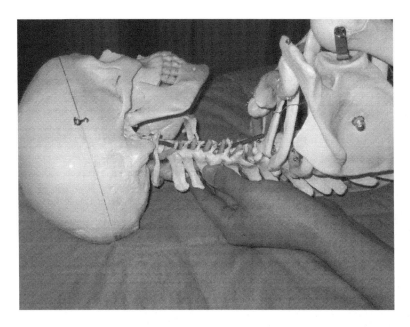

Mastoid Process Cross Fiber work - With fingers, perform a cross fiber stroke on the attachment of the SCM to the Mastoid process. Do slow and steady work in this area, going from anterior to posterior or vice versa depending on directional resistance. The head would stay in neutral position during this stroke, and only one side at a time in order to allow for proper stabilization of your client's head. When working here imagine the 3 dimensions of the SCM at this attachment point. The muscle here is very thick and its surrounding tissue can either move freely or keep the SCM bound to the skull. I've found that working here can bring out many tissue releases that translate into a free moving neck!

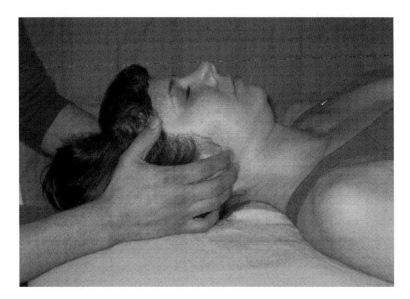

Superficial Anterior Work - Letting your hand become like a bear's paw (meaning, make sure you cover a lot of surface area), bring in a lot of tissue underneath your hand and slowly move towards your client's feet and intend to bring a lengthening and space to the anterior part of their neck area. This is great preparation for anterior neck work. Notice my other hand is supporting my client's head. Another variation to this technique is to bring slight and very slow lengthening to their occiput area as I'm working. My left hand would be moving superiorly as my right hand moves inferiorly or following directional resistance (possibly laterally).

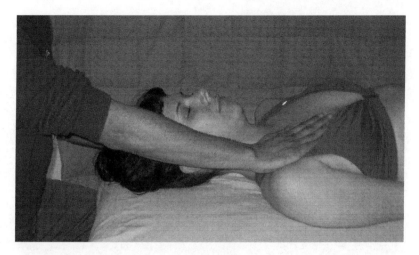

Deeper Work/Anterior Neck Work

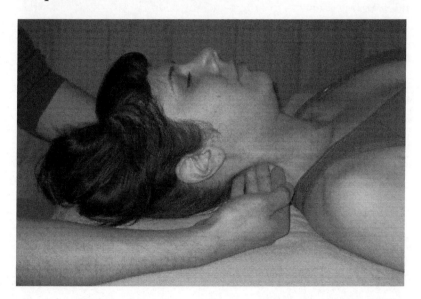

With a couple of fingers, imagine you are peeling away the trapezius from the layer of deeper cervical myo-fascia underneath. You are now working in the posterior triangle area. Doing one side at a time, use your finger pads to do this myo-fascial work. Notice my fingers are close to the client's skull but you can work anywhere along the edge of posterior triangle and even down to where the upper trapezius and the posterior scalene meet. Make sure you slow down enough to sink into that layer between trapezius and deeper cervical myo-fascia. Also remember from this point you can feel the dr of the tissue and go either posteriorly or from superior to inferior directions. Allow the tissue to tell you where to go.

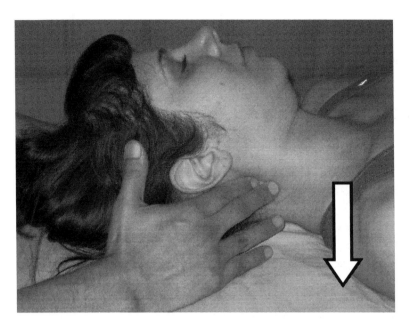

Deeper Scalene Work - Another scalene technique that incorporates the Art Riggs 'Anchor and Lengthen' method is shown here: Sink into the scalenes with your right hand (as shown) while bringing the client's head into flexion with your other hand. Don't strain yourself, it's okay to let the client's head rest on your right hand/wrist. Moving the head in this manner shortens the scalenes (mainly the anterior and middle scalenes) and allows you to sink deeper into its attachments on the ribs.

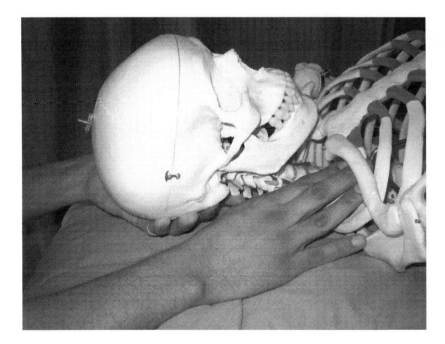

The next picture shows the same picture as before but with a human model. Notice the head is being moved into the direction of the anterior and middle scalene. Once my fingers have sunken into the tissue, I keep my fingers at that level of depth and then slowly bring the client's head back to neutral position. This in effect lengthens the client's scalene muscles. Be aware that this technique can sometimes be intense, monitor your client's reaction to the work and keep open communication about what's happening.

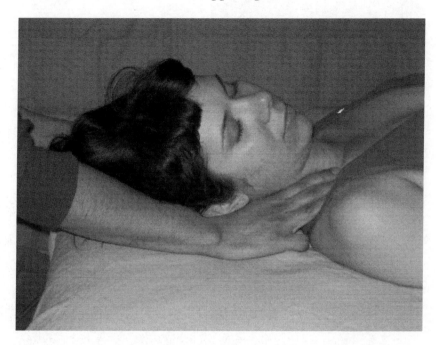

Scalenes in anterior position – In this technique, I am using my left hand and working across the table. I move the Sterno-Cleido Mastoid gently out of the way with my hand. I slowly sink into the layer of tissue medial to the SCM until I find the Scalenes. If you feel a 'thumper' (a pulse), move out of the way. Avoid any direct pressure on any blood vessel. The technique usually ends up moving in a posterior and slightly lateral direction but if you feel directional tightness in a different direction, then follow your palpation sensation.

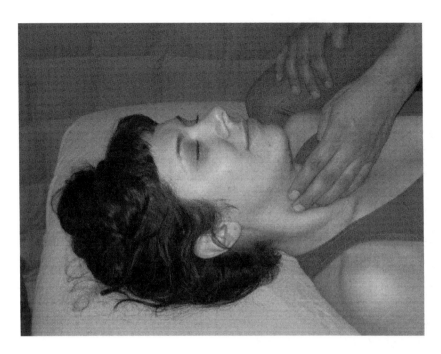

Anterior scalenes in anchor and lengthen method – In addition to sinking into the tissue, you can also sink into the same area (shown from opposite side here) and have the client turn their head towards you. This will lengthen the SCM and access and lengthen anterior muscle/connective tissue. If the client can't rotate their head and instead sidebends, the touch may be too deep or they may not have the articulation to rotate, in which case you may want to attempt an aided rotation technique before-hand.

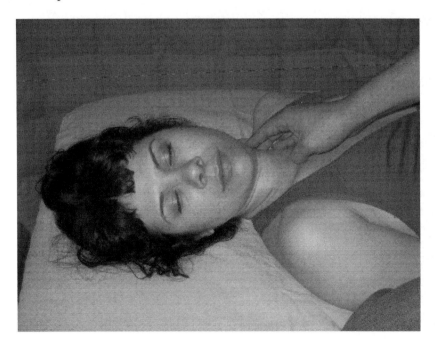

SPINAL MECHANICS

Understanding spinal mechanics is a key step to being able to work on clients with possible vertebrae rotation issues. As this can show up in the context of a series, it's important to deal with these possible issues during a series. If a client is seeing you for neck issues for example and they are in pain, then you may have to work on that first in order to create Adaptability before starting the series. Working on any vertebrae rotation issue can be seen as opening up the energy channel (energy in this case being the force of gravity, tensegrity, greater functionality) that may be necessary to have an effective series. Below are Fryette's laws, which influence spinal mechanics.

FIRST LAW: When the spine is in neutral, side bending to one side will be accompanied by horizontal rotation to the opposite side. What this means is that when you're standing in a neutral position (no bending forward or backward) and you laterally bend/flex or side-bend to the RIGHT for example, your spine will ROTATE to the LEFT (the opposite side). This applies to the thoracic and lumbar vertebrae, the cervical vertebrae (C2 through C7) are the exact opposite of how the thoracic and lumbar behave.

SECOND LAW: When the spine is flexed or extended (non-neutral), side-bending to one side will be accompanied by rotation to the same side. This means that when you flex or extend your spine and you laterally bend/flex or side bend to the RIGHT, your spine will ROTATE to the RIGHT (same side). Again, this refers to the thoracic, lumbar, and C1 vertebrae. The other cervical vertebrae will behave in the opposite manner.

THIRD LAW: When motion is introduced in one plane it will modify (reduce) motion in the other two planes. This is a basic statement about spinal mechanics. When you side bend or forward flex or you do any movement in one plane, there won't be as much motion in the other planes.

In the Morales Method®, we describe vertebral movement as it moves from the VERTICAL AXIS AND FROM THE SUPERIOR POSITION. For example for the lumbar & thoracic spine, if there is a left side-bend in the neutral position, then we expect movement of the vertebra in the Clockwise direction, a product of movement in the sagittal and coronal plane that creates the movement of rotation. When there is a right side-bend in the neutral position, then we expect movement of the vertebra in the Counterclockwise direction for the thoracic and lumbar sections.

The cervical vertebrae from C2 to C7 behave in the opposite manner. When there is a left side-bend of the cervical spine then one or more of the vertebrae will have counterclockwise rotation. When there is a right side-bend, then there will be clockwise rotation.

The following is an example of what can occur in the cervical spine and how the vertebrae and myo-fascial tissue can be involved. Let's take the case of a rotation in the C4 vertebra:

**C4 is rotating CW along the vertical axis (from the superior view) and it's behaving as if it's side-bending to the right.

**SP may be more evident on the left hand side (client in supine).

**Connective tissue may be tense/tight/knotted on left side of SP.

**Directional Resistance may be going in the superior to medial direction on the left side of C4.

**In addition to lengthening tissue in the direction of resistance, we also promote the proper movement of C4 by simultaneously side-bending neck/head to the left, prompting vertebrae to rotate counter-clockwise

CASE STUDY: C4

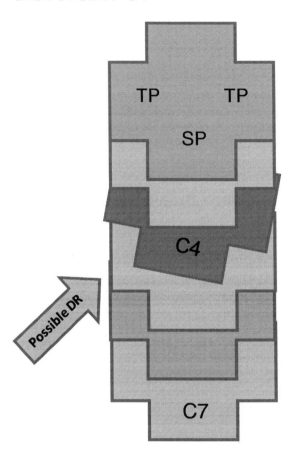

You might notice that a lot of the previous techniques will lengthen tissue such as multifidus and rotatores that may be causing rotation in your client's neck. Aiding in a de-rotation could have already been happening without having to side-bend the client's neck.

The following techniques are meant to assist the practitioner in providing further mobility to a client's neck. Some quick assessment moves that are commonly used beforehand are the checking for ease in side-bending or rotation. Now that you know about spinal mechanics you know what might be happening in your client's neck if they can't look over their left shoulder for example (possible CW rotation of one or more vertebrae?). It's usually not a clear cut case where there's only one vertebrae out of place. It's usually part of a 'symphony of rotation'.

Vertebral facet spacing - With fingers intending to create space between facets, ask client to flex and relax their neck with your fingers in the area between the facets of two vertebrae. This in turn assists to create space between facets while your fingers give the client a cue as to where to flex. Work from C7 to Occiput. You can also focus on one particular set of facets instead of all of them depending on your client's needs. Your fingers should be bent in an angle going superiorly

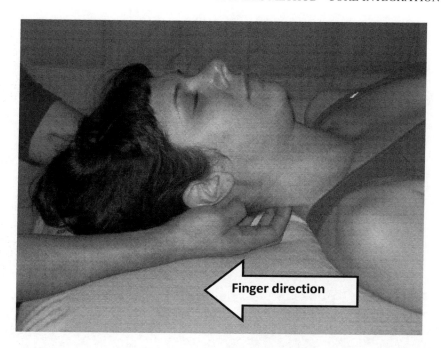

Finger direction

Aided rotation - With one hand, target one vertebra and focus on the soft tissue attached to it. With the other hand move the head into side-bend, nice and slow (remember your spinal mechanics so you know which direction to side-bend) and move them into that side-bend while attempting to work the connective tissue that may be contributing to the rotation. Slow and steady wins the race. If you find a trigger point, you may want to perform trigger point therapy first.

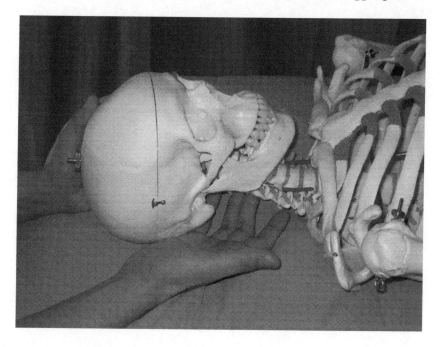

Same technique as above but instead of fingers, use a thumb. Remember the previous technique where your thumb was moving down or up alongside the spinous process. Now we are incorporating side-bending with that technique to assist in vertebral de-rotation.

Note: You can also work going towards the client's head and have your client side-bend on their own as your thumb goes from inferior to superior.

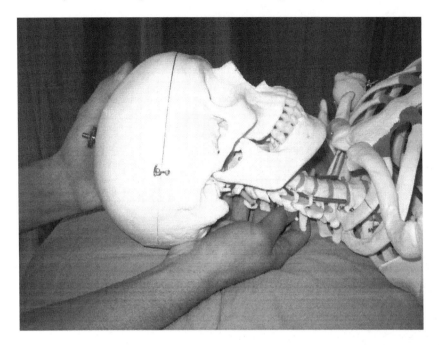

Initiating a de-rotation can also be done by holding the specific vertebrae with one hand that is actually wrapping around the neck and coming from the other direction. In this picture, the skeleton's neck is held and side-bent towards the skeleton's right and the left hand rotates the chosen vertebrae clockwise. My left hand in this case is moving away from the camera and slightly superiorly.

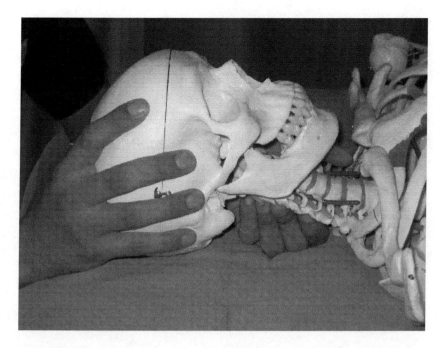

Soft Tissue De-Rotation using multiple planes – To address a side-bend that may be difficult to resolve, you may need to work with the client's neck moving it in multiple planes. The following is a step by step process on how to do that:

1. Address and palpate the rotated vertebrae.

2. With your fingers still in that position, bring the head/neck into flexion. Create a little traction (by striping) to further assist the opening of the facets.

Be aware of your own body mechanics and don't shrug your shoulders.

3. Then bring the head into side-bending range of motion...this aids in de-rotating the rotated vertebrae.

4. Then slowly bring the head into slight rotation, rotating the vertebrae into is proper neutral position. Notice my hands are by the Atlanto-Occipital joint but they can be anywhere depending on which vertebrae is rotated. Go in the reverse direction to finish the technique (rotation then side-bending, then back to neutral from flexion). The client's head is only slightly raised off the table.

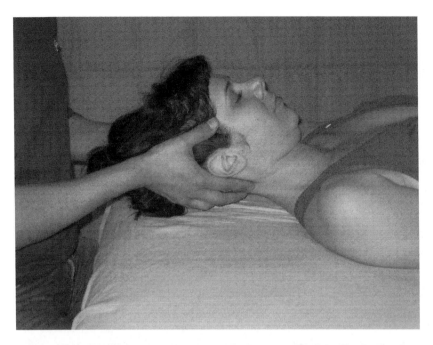

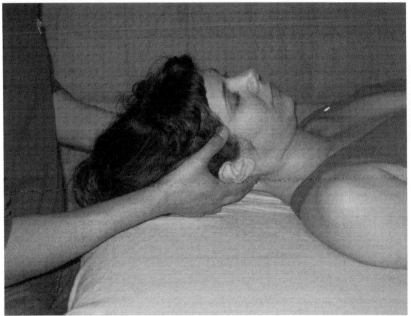

110

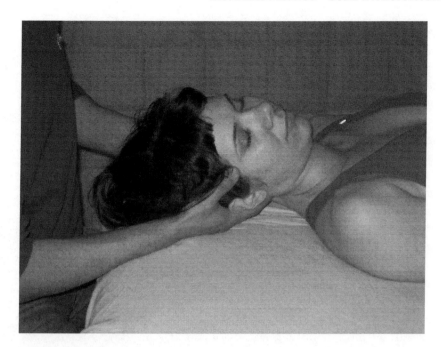

Working the Head

There are so many aspects to working the head but to keep it in a nutshell, the three major muscles or territories you would be dealing with are: Temporalis, Masseter, and Lateral Pterygoid(s). Notice these muscles meet in somewhat the same area. Also note that any tightness/strain from these muscles will affect the very mobile joint that is the TMJ. The following are some notes regarding head and jaw myo-fascial tissue that will affect how we see and work with the head and jaw.

When the External (lateral) Pterygoid muscles contract they pull the top of the mandible closer to the skull. This helps to open the jaw. Tight Lateral Pterygoids can also bring the mandible out of its TMJ. The Pterygoid muscles also help to move the jaw side to side since the mandible is wider than the skull.

The Internal (medial) Pterygoid muscle is similar to the masseter but it is underneath the External (lateral) Pterygoid, attaching to the Pterygoid fossa. Although a Pterygoid, it is more involved with closing the jaw and moving it side to side as opposed to opening the jaw. The coronoid process and zygomatic arch are usually the boney landmarks used to find these muscles.

The Temporalis muscle attaches to (among other places) the area of the jaw close to the last molar tooth, the coronoid process. Again, more convergence in the same area. Think about how tightness in this muscle can lead to pulling the mandible up into the cranium more and could lead to jaw and headaches if that tissue isn't able to relax.

The Masseter inserts onto the mandible and covers the Internal (Medial) Pterygoid. There is actually a major and a minor masseter but we usually work the masseter as a whole.. Again, the masseter aids in closing the jaw.

One way to work the masseter from the outside is to do slow steady work on the masseter major/minor at the ramus of the mandible coming from the zygomatic arch. Moving fingers down towards the mandible. For extra effectiveness have client lower their jaw. Anchor down on the masseter and work it as an 'anchor and stretch' as client raises their jaw. This works the top part of the masseter. Do the opposite move (moving superiorly and asking for opening of the jaw) if you feel the dr calls for it. Another way of working the masseter is to grab it between thumb and forefinger and 'unspiral' the tissue while client has a relaxed jaw. The 'anchor and stretch' technique can also be done with this stroke.

Digastric muscles (again, from the outside) can be worked by working the tissue underneath the mandible. A tight set of digastric muscles can retract the mandible, possibly 'jamming' the mandible into the cranium. Imagine you are scraping the mandible to get to the digastric.

Working the Temporalis can be done in an 'anchor and stretch' method also. One or both can be worked at the same time. Palpate this tissue to see if any areas are 'puffy' or sensitive to the client. I've found that can indicate strain in this myo-fascial tissue. Use 'anchor and stretch' method (holding down where the arrow is as client opens their jaw) or do trigger point therapy on trouble spots. In addition, you can work with the Temporalis 'in movement'. This could mean that your hands move inferiorly as your client slowly opens their jaw. What technique you use will depend on the dr.

For facial muscles, understand that the masseter is underneath most of them. Therefore, working the masseter means you are also working facial muscles and possibly facial nerves so note any type of over sensitivity in the areas you're working on. One of the best ways to know how it feels to do the work is to do the work on yourself. Explore your own face especially around the zygomatic arch and mandible. Realize how it feels to work underneath the arch.

A great book that covers TMJ assessments is Stanley Hoppenfeld's 'Physcial Examination of the Spine and Extremities'. In it you will read about what can happen when your client lowers and raises their jaw and how the mandible tracks if the TMJ is not symmetrical. Do this assessment with yourself in front of a mirror. Does your mandible go straight down? Or does it have a 'curve' in the movement? Remember that if your jaw moves to the left in opening, it's actually the RIGHT hand side lateral Pterygoids that could possibly be tight.

Tight pterygoids (both internal and external) can make the mandible not only open asymmetrically but also in a twisted pattern. Anchor and stretch work can positively affect this pattern. A TMJ that dislocates easily can have a condyle that 'jumps' out & stays out of the groove while the jaw was opening. The condyle usually finds its way back but sometimes it requires re-setting.

Tight Temporalis muscles along with a tight digastric can retract the mandible, again 'jamming' it into the cranium, sometimes causing pain around the ear (sometimes perceived as an earache).

Pterygoids muscles can also bring the jaw out in under-bite style in addition to lowering it (its normal function). If you have a client with this type of jaw, where are the condyles resting and how do the pterygoids feel? Can you see how a client with forward head posture can have a jaw makeup in this same manner?

9 CREATING A SERIES

By now you've seen the structured protocol of a Morales Method® Core Integration Therapy series, gotten a sense of the philosophy behind working in a series, and gotten a perspective of how this system approaches the body. But the big question is: How do we integrate all of this? How would we create a series out of everything we know?

In chapter five I went through what a session would look like. I gave some detail as to how and why I would approach a client with a forward head posture and anterior pelvic shift. The description was only for one session however. To describe nine whole sessions, let's revisit that client and see if we can create a series that revolves around their situation. We will imagine what a client may look like and what some of our strategies might be in working with them. Before we go there, we need to realize this is just one possible scenario and our clients are going to show up with many other variations and possibilities. The scenario constructed here is based on historical patterns and not clinical data. Nevertheless, patterns are important and will help us in addressing clients.
The example: As before, we have a client that is coming in for Morales Method® Core Integration Therapy series work and is exhibiting an anterior shift in their pelvis.
Let's look again at what the hubs could possibly be like:

C1/Skull: Anteriorly shifted
T1/Shoulder Girdle: Posteriorly shifted, rounded shoulders
TL Junction: Posteriorly shifted and tight/locked up
Knees: Possibly posteriorly shifted, over extended
Talus: Anteriorly shifted
Medial Arch: Collapsed
Lateral Arch: Tight

If the client was experiencing pain then the series could actually be twelve sessions, with the first three sessions aimed at helping the client get out of pain and the remaining nine sessions revolving around the series protocol. This is what is meant by Adaptability in this method. If the client was not in pain then the series could follow the nine session protocol. Rather than attempt to spell out all the possibilities that can occur in a session, I will lay out some topics to think about, look out for, and possibly work on in a situation like this. It's very possible that two people with the same type of posture could exhibit different things in their tissue so no two situations are the same. This is what makes this type of work so exciting.

113

Session 1: After seeing the client walk, you may notice a theme to this series. Yes, they are presenting a forward head posture but could it all be dealt with in the head territory or must you keep some other part of their body in mind? Historically the pelvis plays a big part in a forward head posture and it may be the same here. Let's assume the client is posteriorly shifted in their pelvis. Upon further walking you may notice lack of movement in the client's pelvis along the sagittal plane. There may be more movement along the transverse plane but that will be put aside for later as the work in the sagittal plane is the one you want to go for first as it's the most basic plane and should be resolved to first to lay down a proper foundation for functional movement.
1. Check for clockwise or counter clockwise mobility of the tissue around the greater trochanter, that tissue may not be moving in one direction as much as in the other.
2. The gluteal muscles are worked myo-fascially in order to bring more movement along the sagittal plane. Other areas may be seen that need attention that may be limiting sagittal movement. I might work in the plane, possibly working in a superior/inferior direction here.
3. The iliac crest and tissue attached to it could need work to bring sagittal movement there so that area is also palpated and possibly worked while the client is in side-lying position. This is a good positional strategy for this territory.

Afterwards the client may be asked to walk again and we notice if there is more sagittal movement. If so, we would move on to finishing the session. If not, we would address other areas such as the gluteal muscles in prone position, the sacrum and possible sacro-iliac joint restrictions, and the attachments at the ASIS and Ischial tuberosity.
Only once we feel we've adequately addressed the more basic planes keeping in mind the Order of Complexity would we then go to rotation and make sure the client's leg can move in internal or external rotation to its normal degrees of freedom. This could happen in the first session but it could also come up in later sessions (remember, amplitude and the rule of increments).
3. To finish the session and to help with integration of the work, a sacral hold is performed.

Session 2: This session can start either in the leg or the lower leg depending on what is seen in the walking assessment. If it's determined that the lower leg needs the work first and that the territory around the femur has the capacity to receive the changes that will occur below, then session 2 will be a lower leg session. If it's determined via the body reading and assessment that the leg doesn't have the capacity to receive the work that may happen below in the lower leg then you may need to 'build' adaptive capacity by working in the leg (from the knee and above). How do we determine this? One way is to look at the Order of Complexity and see which plane the leg is residing in most when the client walks. If the quadriceps and hamstrings are moving along rotation extensively towards internal rotation (as may happen if the client is knock kneed) then the leg may not be able to accept the work in the lower leg and work on the tissue of the leg (quadriceps, adductors, hamstrings) may need to be done first (within the sagittal plane) to set up the work that will happen in the lower leg.
Let's say this is the case but only slightly, not enough to warrant having to work on the leg first, and we feel the femur territory has the capacity to take on work from below. We will then work the lower leg.
1. If we work on the lower leg we definitely want to make sure there is good Screw Home effect happening in the knee and translating down to the tibia.
2. We also want to make sure there is good tibio-talar joint movement in walking. Some of the

techniques involved in this session could include the standing work to bring more movement to the tibio-talar joint and making sure we address the medial part of that joint.

3. As far as order is concerned, working in the sagittal plane precedes work in rotation so if we want to affect rotation we first want to address ease of movement along the sagittal plane. There are many techniques that could be used for this but I suggest we keep it simple.

We could have our client in supine position and ask them to dorsi-flex their ankle. As they do, I would keep their lower leg in a neutral position and work the tissue that might prevent it from staying in a neutral position. This tissue may be contributing to some rotation but I may initially be working in the sagittal plane since we are following the Order of Complexity.

4. If we didn't have time to work the interosseous membrane (i.o.m.) in session one, then we would work that area now. One way to work it is to sink into an area where the i.o.m. feels restricted, feel for the directional resistance, and take it in the direction of resistance while helping to move the fibula either superiorly or inferiorly by moving the medial malleolus with one hand.

Session 3: If session 2 did not work the leg, then now is the time to do it. Again, we want to continue the work we did in session 2 and we also want to make sure that any work we do in session 3 can be supported by the work done in session 2. Again, if we see a lot of rotation of the femur then we would first work with the sagittal plane to bring ease there first, sort of like priming a pump.

1. Think about asking the client to bring up their knee as if they are going to put their foot on the table. As they do this then I would aid the tissue medially and laterally to the femur to bring that movement in a pure sagittal plane. This would inevitably work some tissue more than other tissue of the quadriceps, adductors, and IT band. My hands act as a guide as the client slowly raises and lowers their knee, adding fluidity to the tissue that is restrictive and aiding in de-rotation of the femur, what we wanted in the first place.

2. Another way to work the sagittal plane would be to work the IT band and feel for directional resistance happening at different areas of the IT band and moving either superiorly or inferiorly.

3. A lot of work usually happens along the sagittal plane; as can be imagined, but think about how the hamstrings can be worked to have them move more efficiently along the sagittal plane. Working the hamstrings with emphasis on the sagittal plane (in the plane) may aid in the balance of rotation of the leg.

Session 4: We are now in the abdominal area. Now that we have worked on the pelvis and have done our best to have it moving in functional balance, we can work the abdominal area so that is moves in conjunction with the pelvis. A lot of emphasis is placed on the psoas in many advanced workshops and trainings (including my own) but we really need to make sure the client is ready to take on psoas work before we go to that core place.

1. How do we make sure there's sufficient movement in the sagittal plane in the abdominal area? We do this by having the client in sideline and checking for how the quadratus lumborum area moves. In this case the lower (inferior) part of the quadratus lumborum tissue is more anterior than the superior part. This may show up as directional resistance, the lower part resisting posterior movement and the upper resisting anterior movement.

2. This territory definitely relates to TL junction and floating ribs but this may need to be addressed in session 5.

3. Address the coronal movement (remember the assessment techniques for the back) of the back tissue, feeling for dr either in clock-wise or counter clock-wise movement.

4. Do the same work on the anterior part, moving the rectus abdominus tissue in both directions. This work is aimed to prepare the client for deeper work in the abdominals

5. Psoas work can be done in conjunction with mesentery work. As with other tissue, make sure the psoas can 'track' well in the sagittal plane before attempting to work with its ability to move transversely. Remember that the work there is to add function/movement in the sagittal plane and my work is tracing that plane.

6. Finally, work with the psoas in its ability to move along rotation, both medial and lateral may occur but keep in mind, this work may not happen in this session if there is so much lack of mobility in the TL junction. Psoas work in rotation may need to occur in a future session.

Session 5: This area covers the TL junction and up to the pectoralis area but does not include scapula. The reason being is that time may need to be dedicated to ribs in this session.

1. In this particular client work will need to be done in the TL junction to encourage mobility in the sagittal plane. Think about putting the client in side-lying position and asking for flexion and then extension right in the TL junction area while working the surrounding tissue feeling for dr.

2. Sometimes this work can be done in standing, asking the client to extend (for example, doing a slight back bend as in the beginning of a Hatha Yoga sun salutation) while we are behind them, working the tissue by the TL junction.

3. Since the pelvis is not as aligned with the ribcage, check the ribs and make sure they are not in a fixed position, either inhalation fixed or exhalation fixed.

4. As with the abdominal area, check the tissue of the superficial back muscles for ease of movement along the coronal plane.

5. Another area that comes to mind is the diaphragm/cartilage territory in the front. An anteriorly shifted pelvis could be related to a closed and tight anterior diaphragm. Work right under the ribcage would be done if restriction was palpated there.

6. Finally, address the pectoralis tissue as it's related to ribs and breath and the work done in the diaphragm will affect the way the top part of the ribcage helps to take in breath.

Session 6: After working the ribcage, we start to address the scapula and the upper ribs as they will relate to the neck. In this particular client this area will exhibit tightness associated to a head that's shifted anteriorly. The scapulae could also be rolled forward, towards the anterior ribcage

1. Work the scapula, with the client in prone, finding the direction of resistance and the direction of ease. With regards to the superior/inferior direction, it will most likely be resistance in the inferior direction (as is often the case) but .

2. From there, work the scapula, moving it in a clock-wise and counter clock-wise manner, feeling for directional resistance in either direction. With a client who has a posterior shift in their shoulder girdle it's possible that the scapulae are protracted so the tissue lateral to it may be short and tight.

3. Special attention is paid to the clavicles here. The clavicles can act as a hub for tissue above and below it and work in the clavicles could be used to create adaptive capacity in the neck area (as the practitioner, you are beginning to do pre-work for session 7).

4. The clavicles are moved in all directions of the coronal plane to feel fro dr and to build ease of movement and to give the client a sense of ease in their shoulder girdle. Remember, if we have opened up the area of the TL junction in previous sessions then the shoulders and clavicles will need to adjust and adapt to the new way of moving.

Session 7: Here we start getting in the home stretch of a series. Although the neck is one of the first places where we as babies start to bring in movement (creating a cervical spine), in a vertical position, as we are in standing, it is one of the last places we work in.

A forward head posture will result in short and tight anterior neck tissue and possibly long and tight posterior neck myo-fascial tissue. This area is not meant to be fully explored early on in the series but if a client has extreme forward head posture then some work early on (remember, the rule of increments) could be done so as not to leave a lot of neck work until the end of the series. Also, remember, working just a bit in the neck before session 7 can build adaptive capacity.

1. One area often ignored in is the most inferior area of the sterno-cleidomastiod (SCM), the place where the SCM meets the clavicle. Creating fluidity and suppleness in this spot helps the neck and head to fully receive the work that was done previously.

2. As we work the neck we need to keep in mind the planes of movement. We would work the neck in this client with respect to sagittal plane first, making sure there is ease of movement in flexion and extension, before we move on to coronal plane movement. Some of the movements previously described will help to bring range of motion in the neck. It's just as important to work along the plane as it is to work in the plane in this territory.

3. Remember the previous techniques regarding the neck and remember the Order of Complexity. We could work the front and back of neck first, then work to bring ease of movement in the side to side movement, aid in the transverse movement of the vertebrae (with special attention to the atlas), and finally, deal with rotation.

Session 8: In this type of structural integration work we separate work in the neck from work in the head and jaw. The reason for this is to allow for adequate time to work with the head and jaw. In our client, it may not be completely evident that there is work to be done in the head and jaw as it is with the client's neck but the work is and the results are what make this work structural integration.

1. Before working inside the jaw work outside the jaw is done, feeling for dr in the sagittal plane in areas such as the temporalis, zygomatic arch, and mandible. If there is a forward head posture than it would be expected to feel resistance in the posterior direction and work would be done accordingly.

2. Working the inside of the jaw includes work on the masseter and the pterygoids. In addition, work on the digastrics is also performed in order to create adaptive capacity for work on the head. Techniques discussed previously encourage movement in the sagittal plane but there are many variations, including work done in sitting and in standing position that help the client create different options for movement.

3. When working the head, imagine the scalp as a cap and feel for the dr of the tissue. Imagine the top of the head as a the top part of a dim sum, where there can be torsion in the tissue that relates to torsions felt down inferiorly. Keeping the Order of Complexity in mind is very important here. If we go straight into de-rotating tissue in the head that seems to be rotated, then we risk leaving something out and encouraging movement that is 'out of sync' with our normal stages of development from our times as a baby, the Order of Complexity.

4. Work in this area can also include work done with the eyes and eye tracking as is done in movement education.

Session 9: This final session is the one done on the arms. Why are arms left until the very end and not done when the scapulae are worked? The answer to this is simple. When looking at the arms, especially the humerus, we notice that it's movement is highly influenced by the movement of the entire body. Any change in the body, even as distant as the talus can have a profound effect on the arm and how we swing it in order to move in our daily lives. We then suppose that if we work the pelvis for example in one session, then work the arm in a subsequent session, and then move back to working the thoracic spine in the session after that, there could be fundamental changes made to the arm that could mean the practitioner would need to go back to the arm again in future sessions. In order to promote efficiency, we therefore leave the arms for last.

Is it possible that this scenario could apply to any part of the body? For example, could the pelvis be affected by work done on the head for example? Yes, that is entirely possible but with the case of the pelvis, it is part of the core as we see it and its relationship with the rest of the core is dynamic. In the case of the arms, its relationship to core is more reactionary (it reacts to what the core wants) and is therefore more at the whim of the core. In that sense, we leave it to the end. There are many aspects to this topic (sensation, athleticism/global movements) that spark many other conversations herein but we will leave those to continue with this series example.

1. We make sure the arm can move in the sagittal plane so we work all tissue around the head of the humerus, typically including rotator cuff tissue. It's very important we cover all tissue that relates the humerus to the scapula and clavicle. Moving the arm along the sagittal plane (without client activation of muscle tissue) will give you information about directional resistance and where to work. Areas often in the repertoire include teres muscles, infraspinatus, and subscapularis.

2. Only after movement in the sagittal plane has been adequately resolved can we move to coronal plane movement and eventually rotation.

3. The bicep/tricep area is a stage for classic movement in the sagittal plane. In this case, the work can be 'in' the sagittal plane (for example working superior/inferior on the bicep or work 'along' the plane (for example on the lateral part of the arm). Eventually rotational work can be done and this work historically addresses mobility at the humeral head at the glenoid fossa. Notice that if rotational work is being done in that spot, then you would have had to make sure work in the pectoral area was done (session 6). This is the logic of the series.

4. The forearm and hand should really deserve their own session but in the interest of time any additional work needed for this area may include a movement session. Structurally, the interosseous membrane is a place addressed and in this session we see the relationships of the radius and ulna here. We also remember that in our session 1 the interosseous membrane comes up as a territory to possibly work as bodyworkers have connected it to core in past trainings.

5. Ideally we wish to see all the functional movement that happens in our client to be accurately expressed in their arms and hands. If we are still running into issues, going back to earlier sessions of the series or including a movement session may be necessary to unlock the reason a client is not moving their arms.

10 CLOSURE

The series ends at the ninth session but work in a series may continue in different forms for a practitioner and client. Among the type of continuation work possible is movement education, as mentioned in chapter 9, to make the work more 'permanent'. Clients often ask, "Will this series 'fix' it once and for all?" to which I explain that one of the main things we are seeking to do as practitioners of Structural Integration is to give the client options for being, options for movement. It is these options that then spark the possibility of being and moving in a different way that is free of pain and discomfort. There is no permanence in this work, only a discovering of more options. Needless to say, movement education is a way to gain more options. This is covered in the actual in person trainings as is the topic of 'homework' and closure work.

When ending a session in this series there may be a couple of minutes spent at the end of a session doing movement work or structural work in a positional strategy other than on the table that may help the client get a different perspective of this additional option being developed in their body. Sometimes it may involve walking behind the client while holding their TL junction area, sometimes it may involve holding a different part of the client as a movement cue while they're walking. Either way, closure at the end of a session is a way for the client to integrate what they've experienced during the session and for them to take the work further as they go on with their day. There are many aspects to this type of work and they are covered in more detail in the actual training.

Recently I was asked a couple of questions about the Morales Method® Core Integration Therapy program by someone considering advanced training. She wrote:

"I'm curious, what prompted you to create your own method of Structural Integration? How does it differ from your Rolf training?

I'm looking forward to learning more about the Morales Method of Structural Integration."

What prompted me to create my own method of SI is not the need for something better but a desire to share with fellow practitioners how my work has changed over the years.
In the beginning my work reflected the classic form of Structural Integration from the Rolf Institute®.

Over the years my work started to change as I included more of my way of seeing things and was influenced by my ongoing training, specifically in motor control learning and neuro motor patterns. What evolved was my own expression of SI, a unique interpretation as I call it. This form of SI made my practice very rewarding so I was determined to share it in hopes of having other practitioners benefit.

I can also answer this question with a quote from Matsuo Basho, "Do not seek to follow in the footsteps of the wise; seek what they sought." The other part of the question can be answered a bit more concretely: Over the years my way of Structural Integration was being influenced by knowledge of motor control development, the work of Art Riggs, and the latest research from many scholars, among them Robert Schleip. This led to an evolution of the way that I work which I started to call Morales Method® Core Integration. It's safe to say Rolfing® and Morales Method® Core Integration are both forms of Structural Integration. So how are they different?

I can sum it up very easily in a few points:
1. First off, the protocol for my method is different from the protocol in Rolfing. This means the territory we work in a Core Integration third session for example is different from the territory worked in a Rolfing third session. The effectiveness of this work lies in my modification of exactly what I originally learned, how I decided to modify it, and then finally how clients reacted to the work. This doesn't mean one protocol is better than another, it just means this derivation has worked for me and that's why I've decided to share it with my fellow practitioners.
2. Secondly, there are 9 basic sessions in a Morales Method® Core Integration series versus the Rolfing® 10 series. With my method there is room for expansion with up to 12 sessions and they are neatly compartmentalized in packets of 3 sessions each.
3. Thirdly, Morales Method® Core Integration Therapy uses a way of working called the Order of Complexity. This Order of Complexity influences everything…how we body read, how we assess, how we work, and the order in which we work. The Order of Complexity is directly derived from the baby stages of motor development and although it may be described differently, this Order of Complexity is used (to some extent) in other modalities, from Feldenkries to SFMA.

You might be asking: Well Marty, if the protocol is different, then how can you be sure that what you're doing is still Structural Integration? This is a great question. Although the protocol is different, the philosophy and the principles that make it Structural Integration are still present in the work and continue to influence the work. Structural Integration can currently be labeled more an art than a science and art is rooted in a way of expression. Both forms of SI share the same path of expression and it gives me great pleasure to see the results of this way of working when bodyworkers discover how to work from a Structural Integration way.

The following is the chart of the Morales Method® Core Integration Program (as of 2016):

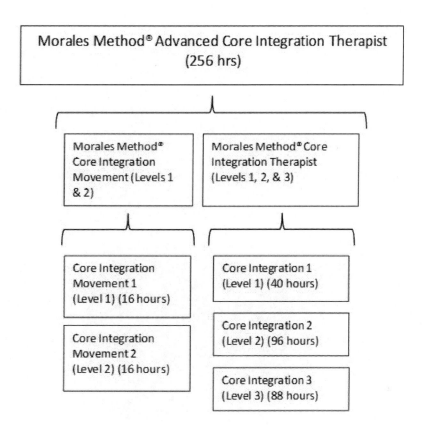

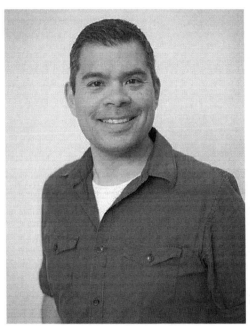

ABOUT THE AUTHOR

Marty Morales, founder of the Morales Method® of Manual Therapy and Body Conditioning, Certified Advanced Rolfer™, and MBA has been practicing in California and teaching students throughout the U.S. and internationally for the past decade. Based in San Francisco, California, Marty has enjoyed bringing his way of working to students throughout the world and helping thousands of people live pain free lives. A published author, Marty has written "Mastering Body Mechanics - A Visual Guide for Bodyworkers", now in its second edition, and has written numerous articles.

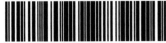

Made in the USA
San Bernardino, CA
17 November 2017